Reset Your Thyroid:

21-day Meal plan to reset your thyroid

To jumpstart your weight loss success

You will find in this book intensely flavorful recipes that are delicious, easy to make that are simply wonderful and will make your taste buds scream with delight.

This book thanks everyone suffering from hypothyroidism and looking for answers. And for all the nutritionists, holistic health professionals and medical professionals who are making a difference in the field of nutrition and hypothyroidism. A lack of knowledge is a lack of power.

Your Personal Contract

I..

Declare that I will master my life in every aspect of it. I will no longer settle for less than I deserve. I have the courage, will power and wisdom to know that it's my time to make a difference in my life. I will put my best foot forward in all areas of my life. I will wake up grateful, put the right foods in my body for nourishment and uplift others.

I am the only person responsible for my life and I believe with every fiber of my being that that I can make a difference.

I am enough. I will be true to myself and follow my heart. My personal development is in my own hands AND I will stop fighting against myself. I will stop listening to self-doubt. My past experiences will not affect my current mindset. God will support me in with joyful abundance in all areas of my life. This book is only the beginning of my wonderful journey to happiness, joy, peace and prosperity. I am willing to go beyond my past and I am the only person who chooses my path and I don't need anyone's approval. I release all limitations from my past.

I will seek the highest truth and the most healing ways to live my life. Health and Happiness is abundantly mine.

Love,

Signed by ....

Disclaimer

The information and recipes contained in book are based upon the research and the personal experiences of the author. Every attempt has been made to provide accurate, up to date and reliable information. No warranties of any kind are expressed or implied. Readers acknowledge that the author is not engaging in the rendering of legal, financial, medical or professional advice. By reading this book, the reader agrees that under no circumstance the author is not responsible for any loss, direct or indirect, which are incurred by using this information contained within this book. Including but not limited to errors, omissions or inaccuracies. This book is not intended as replacements from what your health care provider has suggested. The author is not responsible for any adverse effects or consequences resulting from the use of any of the suggestions, preparations or procedures discussed in this book. All matters pertaining to your health should be supervised by a health care professional. I am not a doctor, or a medical professional. This book is designed for as an educational and entertainment tool only. Please always check with your health practitioner before changing your diet, taking any vitamins, supplements, or herbs, as they may have side-effects, especially when combined with medications, alcohol, or other vitamins or supplements. Please check with you health care provider to see if you can switch to a hypothyroidism diet whereas you might have other health conditions that will not allow you to. Knowledge is power, educate yourself and find the answer to your health care needs. Wisdom is a wonderful thing to seek. I hope this book will teach and encourage you to take leaps in your life to educate yourself for a happier & healthier life. You have to take ownership of your health. All rights reserved. No part of this publication may be reproduced, distributed, or transmitted in any form or by any means, including photo copying, or recording, or other electronic, or mechanical methods, without the prior written permission of the author, except in the case of brief quotations, embodied in critical reviews, in certain other noncommercial uses permitted by copyright laws. Although every precaution has been taken by the author to verify the accuracy of the information contained herein, the author assumes no responsibility for any errors, or omissions. No liability is assumed for damages that may result from the information that is obtained within.

A.L. Childers

Copyrighted Material

Copyright 2016 Audrey Childers.

This book, or parts thereof, may not be reproduced in any form without the written permission from the Author. All rights reserved. This book is copyright protected. You cannot sell, distribute, use, quote or paraphrase any part or the content within this book without of the author. Legal action will be pursued if breached.

All rights reserved. In accordance with the U.S. write copyright act of 1976, the scanning, the uploading, and electronic scanning of any part of this book. Without permission of the publisher or author constitutes unlawful piracy and theft of the author's intellectual property. If you would like to use material from this book. (Other than for review purposes), prior written permission must be obtained by contacting the author @ permissions @ audreychilders@hotmail.com. Thank you for your support of the author's rights.

Thanks for reading my latest book. Please let me know if you need any support with it.

Introduction:

Around 20 million Americans and 250 million people worldwide will be affected by low thyroid function or hypothyroidism. One in 8 women will struggle with a thyroid problem in her lifetime, and up to 90% of all thyroid problems are autoimmune in nature, the most common of which is Hashimoto's. Many people don't know that hypothyroidism is an autoimmune disease and the reason why most doctors don't mention is because it's simple: it doesn't affect their treatment plan. Traditional medicine treats autoimmune disorders with steroids and other methods that suppress the immune system. The number of people suffering from hypothyroidism continues to rise each year. Levothyroxine is the 4th highest selling drug in the U.S. Every Cell in your body responds to your thyroid hormones. These hormones have a direct impact on every major system in your body.

Hypothyroidism is the kind of disease that carries a bit of mystery with it. This book is not for readers looking for quick answers. There is not one size fits all. You have to be in charge of your health. I didn't write this book to sell you any "snake oil" in a bottle. I've written this book to be an eye opener for you and to share with you what I have learned on my journey. The solutions in this book has helped so many people. There are many incredible holistic practitioners, authors and researchers with experience and expertise in this area. I've done my best to pull from all their expertise, as well as my own knowledge and clinical experience. I want to make it easy for you to find the answers quickly, all in the one place, because I'm all too familiar with that awful side effects of hypothyroidism. I certainly don't want you to have to spend years finding solutions, like I did. I also what you to understand that there isn't an easy "one pill" solution, but the "one pill" approach that our current medical system is using is NOT WORKING because the underlying cause for hypothyroidism is not being addressed. Many people never question their doctors, research their medications or find out the side effects of what was prescribed. Don't misconstrue what I am saying being on medication isn't a bad thing when it is necessary but sometimes the medications that are given will camouflage the real symptoms. The problem with giving people thyroid hormone is that it may not be addressing the root cause of your hypothyroidism. If you start addressing the root cause your body will start to heal itself. All these years of bad eating habits beginning in your childhood, a stressful life, lack of exercise/too much exercise, environmental toxins and little to no sleep have contributed to your hypothyroidism. So many of us have these crazy phantom-like health problems. The best patient to be is a well informed and an educated patient. This book can make the difference between you having the energy to live your life as you want, or merely dragging yourself through life. Don't be upset with your medical doctor or endocrinologist they are there to treat your illness not really to give advice on getting to the root of the cause. These doctors are needed. A Health Practitioner will get to the root of your cause and start helping you heal yourself from the main underlying issues. In this book, you will learn the link that ties many of our issues together. Get ready to go on a journey of discovery where you are going to learn how everything ties into one. The foods we eat can interfere with your thyroid medication. Our body is lacking certain nutrients that heavily influence the function of our thyroid gland while certain foods can inhibit your body's ability to absorb the replacement hormones. There is no one size fits all program when you are dealing with hypothyroidism. When you start to eat smarter and are aware of what foods feed your body, despite the condition, you can start to feel better and manage your symptoms. In this age of overly processed, genetically modified, artificially flavored and preservative loaded foods. I'm very excited that you bought this book and are wanting to find an answer to what is hindering your life. Think about this. Americans are in such a pathetic health crisis. We have the abundance of everything at our finger tips but yet we 1 in 3 people are on some sort of medication. It doesn't matter if it's Prescribed or over the counter. Meanwhile billions of people around the world are in better health than the average American, doesn't have to be on some sort of medication and are in their correct body mass index. We are in such a state of denial. My mission is to do everything in my power to help you to start healing and reach your fullest potential. To help be a source of inspiration you seek and attract what you desire with the faith that your vision of success is your destiny! You deserve to kick yourself out of that fat storage unhealthy mode and into a fat burning healthy mode. Remember, what we eat, governs what we become.

A note of caution:

I strongly support self-care, personal health empowerment and improving your understanding of thyroid health. However, this cannot substitute by a trained medical professional in cases of long standing and undiagnosed symptoms. This book is thus not meant as a substitute for professional medical judgement, though it can serve as a helpful adjunct to it.

When in doubt about your thyroid seek your doctor or your medical professional to exclude serious medical conditions.

Be safe, be sane and be healthy.

Get a complete exam from a reliable health practitioner. Do what you can do within the boundaries of good common sense.

In a word, be kind to yourself and your thyroid.

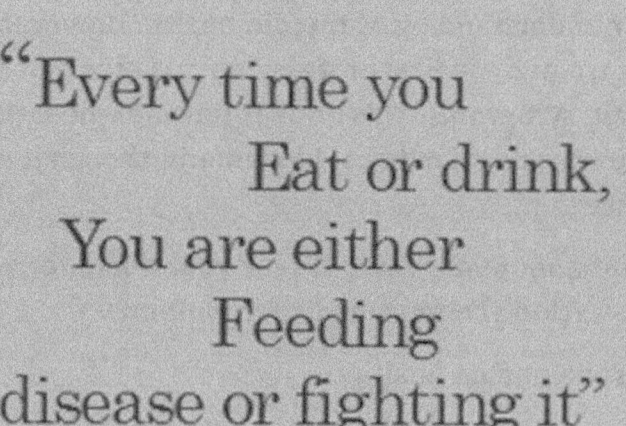

"Every time you Eat or drink, You are either Feeding disease or fighting it"

Author Note:

Let's not forget that we are all different. Each one of us are unique and we are biochemically individually wired and what works for one person may not work for another. We are extremely complex and each person should be valued independently. My reason for having hypothyroidism might not be your reason. Hypothyroidism isn't a 1 size fits all solution. I want to try to help you understand the many debilitating aspects of this medical condition. This book is packed full of repetitive information and is meant to be an eye opener for everyone who wants to make a difference in their lives and what some doctors just won't tell you. I want this book to be just one of your resources that is empowering to try to help you make sense of it all. We need our medical doctors, health practitioners and those who have studied years but I urge you to also find another doctor if your doctor won't listen to you or even allow you to see your lab results or even if you doctor refuses to perform necessary needed lab work.

You must realize that the thyroid has a relationship with all the hormones. It's a very complex balance and there is no straight forward treatment of just treating your thyroid alone. Everyone is different it isn't an easy one size fits all task.

DISCOVER YOUR POSSIBILITES

I've worked really hard with these recipes and I know we all have different tastes but I certainly hope that you like these recipes and enjoy them as much as I do. Please feel free to mix and match any and all recipes. You can have breakfast for dinner and a dinner for breakfast. This is your journey. So, what are you going to eat? This might have been your first thought when you started on your discovery after being diagnosed with Hypothyroidism. I've put together a sample 21 day meal plan as a way of sharing with you some of the many delicious possibilities while you start on your new adventure. Here are a few tips to get you started:

Embrace Yourself

Since it takes 21 days to form a new habit, it will most likely take that long for your mind and body to stop opposing your new lifestyle change. Three weeks really isn't a very long time. If you find yourself in a rut and coming up with excuses. You can regain control by reminding yourself that you only have to do it for 21 days. Motivate yourself to exercise. Choose something you honestly like to do and won't loathe at least 3 times a week. Create an exercise plan that seems easy to accomplish. (And, stick to it!) Give yourself a chance and commit to yourself to stay with the program for 21 days.

Eat What You Need

  Your body is unique. Be mindful of how you eat. Eat slowly, enjoy every mouthful, and think about what you're eating. Drink plenty of water. Take your body weight and divide it by two. That is how many ounces a day you need to consume. Always strive for no less than 8 glasses of 8 ounces of filtered water per day. Try your best to get 7 hours of sleep each day, practice breathing technique and meditate. If you find yourself at a breaking point , to help get your mind off of your body change, try to simplify your home or office space (such as spending 15–20 minutes daily cleaning out and organizing drawers, closets, and cupboards) , read a new book, walk, talk to a friend. Keeping yourself busy can help you forget about those negative health- and life-destroying habits that you are trying to overcome. If you need more encouragement visit my Facebook page Hypothyroidism Healing and Support by Audrey. I am here to support you.

Realize you're Not Alone

Beware of negative self-talk. Sometimes we can be our worst enemy. We convince ourselves that we are not good enough, not smart enough, no pretty enough, not tall enough, not thin enough, not wealthy enough, the list can keep going. Don't give in to that voice. Mute all the mental negative voices that whisper lies to you. Every one of us is unique. We all need to push away all of societies labels, stigmas and stereotypes attached to women. God made you for a reason. You are beautiful. Your greatness is limitless, but to achieve this, 1st you must believe in yourself.

The 21 Day Reset

Changing your habits to become a better you.

One of the most inspiring facts about life is that it flows from the inside out. We're affected by what happens inside—our feelings and our thoughts— our health and our happiness all of these things play a very important role in how see view the world every day. This has a direct impact on our well-being, it can change our mindset, the words we convey, and our response with the world. We've all heard that our gut is called the "second-brain". Given how closely the two interact with each other one thing you may not realize is your emotions and weight gain can start in the gut. Your gut and digestion can also cause you to hold onto that excess weight and just feel lousy. I know, you've heard that it takes 21 days to form a new habit.

The shocking truth is YOU have the power.

I've been battling hypothyroidism for years. After many unsuccessful doctors' appointments over the years, it seemed none offered me ideas on diet change. It was here take this pill. I decided that I had to take charge of my health. You have to heal your body from the inside out. My goal in life is to share my knowledge of what has worked for me.

I've written 9 books in total about hypothyroidism. Each book goes in depth and they all hit different areas and angles of this serious and most often debilitating condition. You can find them all on Amazon. All my books are filled with powerful knowledge and unprocessed recipes that will refuel-your-body, supercharge your metabolism, revitalize thyroid function, and help you shed those excess pounds! Along with bonus recipes for natural body recipes and nontoxic house cleaning ideas. It's not about being skinny, it's about gaining energy, vitality, and feeling good when you look in the mirror." I hope you become inspired." Please check out my blogs @ Thehypothyroidismchick.com.

You're worth it.

I have complete faith in you. I want to challenge you to make a promise to yourself to take the 21 day step. I have given you the blueprint of what you need to do to achieve extraordinary results. The reason for this book is to help you reach your fullest potential. You are going to kick your body out of fat storage mode and into a fat burning mode.

Make a habit of believing in things most people think are impossible. Learn to question everything. Experts will always try to convince you that what you want to do is impossible and simply won't work. However, every successful endeavor starts with one stubborn person who refuses to operate by the same rules and type of thinking that everyone else does. Be that person." - Mark MacDonald, Co-CEO and Co-Founder of Appster

Life

Success is getting what you want. Happiness is wanting what you get.

Stop surviving and start thriving.

Sometimes your life just needs clarity. You have to step out of your comfort zone and focus on what your heart desires. If you desire to be healthier, happier or have a more fulfilled life then you need to take the steps necessary to achieve those goals. No one is going to do this better than you. No one will do this for you. You were born with the capacity of abundance. You have to clear away any of the emotional, mental, and energetic debris that is in the way of your ability to see who you really are and create the life you really deserve. Right now, you are making different choices. You deserve to this! The journey has just begun. Congratulations. You've taken your 1st steps into becoming a more beautiful you. I challenge you to find your inner strength. Focus on that vision and get a clear picture of what you want. Speak words of inspiration to your soul. Say things like, "I will do things to make a difference in my health", "I am beautiful", "I am happy". I am not going to sugar coat this it does take some work. You're unstoppable. Life is the ultimate adventure. Every day we are filled the opportunities to make an impact and have a ripple effect on our health and others around us. Be the Spark! I thank you for being curious and seeking after the truth. All of us, who were told it was all in our head, all of us who wouldn't take no for the answer and demanded a change. No more being stuck in limbo and feeling like you can't get out of this rut. You will make a difference not only in your health but the health and well-being of others. You have the power and you have the mindset.

3 things that you can do to shift your mindset. When you feel bombared with life and things are not going your way. Stop , take a deep breathe, and write down on a piece of paper. Yes, I am going old school. Pen and paper.

1. What do you have that makes you grateful?
2. What do you love and why?

Don't just list what you love and are grateful for. List why . Embelish them. Bask in them. Be specific why you appreciate it.

3. Be grateful for for the small mercies in life.

Only when you open your eyes with gratitude the you can honestly see the world for what it is. It is a beautiful thing!

If you compare your elf to others , please, stop that revolving door of comparison and negativity. Surround yourself with people who don't value YOU, on your looks but your heart and self worth.

Become SOUL FOOD!

Be someone who brings value to other's lives. Someone who lifts others up when they are down. Someone who doesn't judge. Someone who looks for beauty beyond skin deep.

Which do you think would make you feel happy, valuable, and whole?

We have been programmed since birth by the world around us on how we look. Especially as women, we play the "comparison" game with all the celebrity and supermodel bodies while we are swamped with in social media, tv programs and movies.

I a guilty of playing the "comparison" game with how I looked, and I have been in situations in the past that truly made me feel like I was "eye candy." My heart didn't matter, MY goals didn't matter, and MY opinion didn't matter.

So what happened to me while I was obsessed and worried about how I look? Stress, Sadness, Self-sabotage... All bad things..

Beauty radiates from the inside -out.

Become SOUL FOOD!

> If you always do what you always did, you will always get what you always got.
>
> — Albert Einstein

Hypothyroidism means your thyroid is not making enough thyroid hormone. Your thyroid is a butterfly-shaped gland in the front of your throat. It makes the hormones that control the way your body uses energy. Basically, our thyroid hormone tells all the cells in our bodies how busy they should be. Our bodies will go into overdrive with too much thyroid hormone (hyperthyroidism) and our bodies slow down with too little thyroid hormone (hypothyroidism). The most common causes of hypothyroidism worldwide is dietary and environmental. The most common cause of hypothyroidism is dietary and environmental! What does that mean exactly? That means you need to be eat to cater to your thyroid and stop using all these harmful chemicals to clean your home with and put on your body!

It's not hard. Yes, a little adjustment will be needed but isn't everything we do in life for the better of our health worth a little inconvenience until it becomes a habit?

Here are a list of symptoms that Hypothyroidism can cause:

Dry skin and brittle nails

Your fingertips becoming numb

Feeling fatigued, weak, or depressed

Constipation

Memory problems or having trouble thinking clearly

Heavy or irregular menstrual periods

Joint or muscle pain

Dry skin

Hair loss

Headaches

Unexplained weight gain

Thinning hair

Clammy palms

Difficulty swallowing

Sensation of lump in throat

Dry, itchy scalp

Diminished sex drive

Persistent cold sores, boils, or breakouts

Elevated levels of LDL (the "bad" cholesterol)

Heightened risk of heart disease

Heart Palpitations

Dry skin and brittle nails

Your fingertips becoming numb

Feeling fatigued, weak, or depressed

Constipation

Memory problems or having trouble thinking clearly

Heavy or irregular menstrual periods

Joint or muscle pain

Unexplained weight gain

Difficulty swallowing

Sensation of lump in throat

Dry, itchy scalp

Diminished sex drive

Persistent cold sores, boils, or breakouts

Elevated levels of LDL (the "bad" cholesterol)

Heightened risk of heart disease

Heart Palpitations

Inability to lose weight

Inability to eat in the mornings

Tightness in throat; sore throat; horse sounding voic

Hypothyroidism Diet

Here is a list of foods that are in aboundance that will be and won't be on your plate during your journey.

Foods to eat!

I'm not going to sugar coat this program. Eating healthy is hard but it's worth every mouthful! Two area's in this book, I will list things that will help you heal from the inside out. Foods that are dense in nutrients. You can eat hormone free chicken, hormone free turkey, duck, whole eggs, grass fed meats, wild game, shrimp, crab, lobster, wild Alaskan salmon, wild-fish sardines, trout and herring. You want to go for foods that are good for your thyroid, anti-inflammatory and low on the G.I. chart. Parsley, ginger, onions, romaine lettuce, scallions, shallots, asparagus, garlic, green beans , artichokes, carrots, green peas, sweet corn, mushrooms, tomatoes, chilies, red, orange and green bell peppers, apples , apricots, prunes, oranges, kiwi, coconut, coconut milk, cherries, red grapefruit, brown rice, dark chocolate, yam, sweet potatoes, rolled oats, hummus, walnuts, chick peas, kidney beans, butter beans, navy beans, lentils, black eye pea's, yellow split peas, organic apple cider vinegar, celery, cinnamon, cucumber, flax seed, squash, zucchini, green tea, lemons , limes, hot sauce, pineapple , pumpkin, red wine, quinoa, wild rice, turmeric, ghee butter, coconut oil, coconut amino's. Fresh fruits and vegetables as snack are always encouraged. Apples, apricots, prunes, oranges, kiwi, cherries, red grapefruit, plums and pineapple. These are good for your thyroid fruits!

Foods to limit!

Cruciferous Vegetables

Cruciferous vegetables are a great source of fiber, are rich in nutrients, carotenoids, vitamins C, E, and K; folate, antioxidants and minerals. There hasn't been any known human study that has demonstrated a deficiency in thyroid function from consuming a unlimited amount of cooked cruciferous vegetables. However, there has been a known case report to where an 88-year-old woman developed severe hypothyroidism and went into a coma after consuming an estimated 2-3 lbs of raw bok choy every day for several months. In fact, cruciferous vegetables protect against thyroid cancer and has many anti-cancer benefits. Cruciferous vegetables are rich sources of sulfur-containing compounds known as glucosinolates. Some glucosinolates found in raw cruciferous vegetables produces a compound known as goitrin, which has been found to interfere with thyroid hormone production. Very high intakes of raw cruciferous vegetables, such as raw cabbage and raw turnips, have been found to cause hypothyroidism. If someone developed hypothyroidism from consuming large amounts of cooked cruciferous vegetables. I would suggest that they have their iodine checked and don't forget everything in moderation. Limit your intake of cooked cancer fighting veggies to a few times a week but please eat your cancer fighting veggies. The benefits clearly outweigh the risks.

- Arugula
- Bok choy
- Broccoli
- Brussels sprouts
- Cabbage
- Cauliflower
- Chinese cabbage
- Collard greens
- Daikon radish
- Mustard greens
- Radish
- Rutabaga
- Shepherd's purse
- Turnip
- Watercress
- Kohlrabi
- Landcress

Horseradish   kale

Let's go over some important things. We are one of the richest country in the world and we have an abundance of food everywhere it seems but yet we are extremely malnourished and mineral deficient. Why is that? We are literally starving our bodies to death. How can this be? Our problem is that even with all of this abundance of food , readily available at our hands, people aren't obtaining the basic nutrients their bodies needs in order to fuel what is needed to perform the necessary basic functions. The Standard American diet in a nutshell of unhealthy saturated fats and Trans fats, our meals are unbalanced, oversized, and loaded with cholesterol, salt, sugar, artificial ingredients and preservatives. There is about 20 million estimated Americans have some form of thyroid disease. Women are five to eight times more likely than men to have thyroid problems and one woman in eight will develop a thyroid disorder during her lifetime.

Facts about the Thyroid Gland and Thyroid Disease

The thyroid is a hormone-producing gland that regulates our body's metabolism— it affects our major body functions for example your heart rate and energy levels. The thyroid gland determines the rate in which your body produces the energy from nutrients and oxygen. The thyroid gland is located in the middle of the lower neck.

Although the thyroid gland is relatively small, it produces a hormone that influences every cell, tissue and organ in the body. Imagine that!

Hypothyroidism is a condition where the thyroid gland does not produce enough thyroid hormone. A few of the many symptoms are extreme fatigue, depression, forgetfulness, and some weight gain.

We need to change the way we eat. If we are what we eat what would you be made up of? We need to change the chemicals we use on our bodies and change the chemicals we use in our homes. We have to get back to clean eating. Eat to feed your thyroid. Could it be that simple? I think, so YES! Chemicals, additives and GMO foods are added to most of all the foods that are readily and easily available on every supermarket shelves. We are so unaware of the things that are added to our foods like hormones, antibiotics, plastics, extra chemicals, addictive's, cancer causing preservatives, dyes, coloring agents and why? Why would our FDA allow this to go on? To continue slowly poisoning us. Why do we trust the FDA and take a chance on our health, our livelihood and our future?

Here are a few quick tips to jump start your hypothyroidism health!

1. **Adopt a Healthy Diet, Avoid Gluten**

Your thyroid is depending on your to start feeding it and start maintaining your overall health. So stick with whole, natural, and organic foods. Steer clear of processed foods and eat gluten free. Gluten can have undesirable effects on the thyroid.

2. **Avoid Soy**

Soy products have hormone disrupting effects. Soy is also high in isoflavones (or goitrogens), which can damage your thyroid gland. Products containing soy protein appear in nearly every aisle of the supermarket. That's because soy doesn't just mean tofu. Traditional soy foods also include soymilk, soynuts and edamame (green soybeans), just to name a few. Food companies also develop new food products containing soy protein from veggie burgers to fortified pastas and cereals. READ your labels. Don't worry you still can eat fried brown rice but replace it with Coconut amino's instead.

3. Iodine

Iodine is a very popular hypothyroidism natural treatment source and many natural health experts do recommend a good source of iodine. While nascent iodine is most often recommended, Lugol's brand is a fine alternative. Dr. Group's iodine supplement, is also a viable option. Vitamins C and E, D3, selenium and zinc, and omega-3s should be supplemented with your choice of iodine as well.

Some food sources of iodine include:

- Seaweed and sea vegetables
- Some yogurts (organic yogurt, Greek)
- Cranberries
- Strawberries

- Dairy products
- Dulse flakes

Keep in mind that many hypothyroidism cases are actually caused by Hashimoto's thyroiditis. It was found in some research that increasing iodine intake could actually cause your thyroid issues to worsen if you have Hashimoto's. Instead, reducing iodine intake may be the solution.

4. Eat More Antioxidant-Rich Foods

Antioxidants are also important in keeping your thyroid healthy. But rather than getting them from traditional multivitamins, that simply exit the body just as easily as they entered, obtain them from natural food sources. Load up on vitamin C from dark green vegetables and citrus fruits, Omega 3 fats from walnuts and flax seeds, and zinc from pumpkin seeds.

5. Reduce Exposure to the Chemical PFOA (Found in Non-Stick Cookware)

Finally, reduce your exposure to PFOA, found in common household products including nonstick cookware and waterproof fabrics. Researchers have found that people with higher levels of PFOA (perfluorooctanoic acid) have a higher incidence of thyroid disease. Start cooking with cast iron skillets or stainless steel cookware.

6. Coconut Oil

Raw, Virgin Coconut oil has been used as just one hypothyroidism natural treatment. Coconut oil is made up of medium chain fatty acids known as medium chain triglyceride's (MCTs), which help with metabolism and weight loss, coconut oil can also raid basal body temperatures – all good news for people suffering from low thyroid function.

7. Natural Hormone Balancing

One approach to fixing thyroid issues and hypothyroidism is the use of hormone therapy. You really need to meet with a holistic expert. There are many great holistic and naturopath doctors. Most often, synthetic hormones like Synthroid, Levoxyl, or Levothroid are used, which contain only the T4 hormone and no T3 – two hormones produced by the thyroid gland. Thyroid conditions can be serious. You should always seek a professional who knows how to help you. Our organs and glands like your thyroid, adrenals, pituitary, ovaries, testicles and pancreas regulate most of your hormone production, and if your hormones become even slightly imbalanced it can cause some serious health issues. Our gut health can also play an important role in hormone regulation. Start loading up on up on rich sources of natural omega-3s like wild fish, flaxseed, chia seeds, walnuts and grass-fed animal products. People don't boost their omega-3 foods intake to balance out the elevated omega-6s they consumed. To many mega-6 foods will cause inflammation and lead to chronic disease. Eating more coconut oil, salmon, grass fed butt like Ghee and avocados will start to provide your body with essential fats that are fundamental building blocks for hormone production. Supplements like digestive enzymes, probiotics, bone broth, kefir, fermented vegetables, and high-fiber foods can start to repair your gut lining, which also can help to balance your hormones. Caffeine will rise your cortisol levels and then it lowers your thyroid hormone levels and basically creates havoc throughout your entire body. Replace your morning coffee with herbal teas. Matcha tea is a great caffeine replacement and is loaded with antioxidants, weight loss benefits, and cancer fighting properties, heart health, brain power, skin health and a good Chlorophyll Source. Last but not least

GET OUT IN THE SUN! Free vitamin D, baby. 20 minutes a day is a great way to soak up some that free essential vitamin. On the days where you can't sit out in the sun you can supplement with a good D3 vitamin.

8. Foods that you should start incorporating in your everyday eating.

Figuring out how much you need to eat for you own unique body will require time and experimentation. Eat slowly and mindfully until you are 80% full. You want to feel satisfied but not stuffed. If you exercise more, you need more calorie intake. You can easily start with a salad and add more veggies, healthy, fats and proteins to any meal. You need to make sure you're getting enough nutrients per day. Try your best to not eat 3 hours prior to bedtime and after your last meal allow a 10 hour window before you eat again. How you use food is a way to you can do to start naturally balancing your hormones in your kitchen.

9. Beneficial bacteria supports your immune system

For most people, taking a quality probiotic supplement doesn't have any side effects other than higher energy and better digestive health. As a society we have drastically cut back on our consumption of vegetables and of beneficial essential fatty acids (flax, pumpkin, black current seed oil, dark green leafy vegetables, hemp, chia seeds, fish) such as those found in certain fish (including salmon, mackerel, and herring) and flaxseed. We are consumed with little fiber and an excess of sugar, salt, and processed foods. Stress, changes in the diet, contaminated food, chlorinated water, and numerous other factors can also alter the bacterial flora in the intestinal tract. When you treat the whole person instead of just treating a disease or symptom, an imbalance in the intestinal tract stands out like an elephant in the room. So to play it safe, I recommend taking a probiotic supplement every.

Probiotics are live bacteria and yeasts that are good for your health, especially your digestive system. Probiotics are often called "good" or "helpful" bacteria because they help keep your gut healthy. Probiotics foods include yogurt, kefir, Kimchi, Sour Pickles (brined in water and sea salt instead of vinegar) Pickle juice is rich in electrolytes, and has been shown to help relieve exercise-induced muscle cramps., Kombucha, kombucha tea ,Fermented meat, fish, and eggs.

Prebiotics foods are brown rice, oatmeal, flax, chia, asparagus, Raw Jerusalem artichokes, leeks, artichokes, garlic, carrots, peas, beans, onions, chicory, jicama, tomatoes, frozen bananas, cherries, apples, pears, oranges, strawberries, cranberries, kiwi, and berries are good sources. Nuts are also a prebiotic source.

The ideal pH for the colon is very slightly acidic, in the 6.7–6.9 range. When there is an imbalance or lack of beneficial bacteria in the colon, the pH is typically more alkaline, around 7.5 or higher. The optimal pH range for gas-producing organisms is slightly alkaline at 7.2–7.3.

When someone starts taking a probiotic or a prebiotic supplement (or eats a prebiotic food), the beneficial microorganisms begin to increase in number. These good bacteria start to ferment more soluble fiber into beneficial products like butyric acid, acetic acid, lactic acid, and propionic acid. These acids provide energy, improve mineral, vitamin, and fat absorption, and help prevent inflammation and cancer. The extra acid also starts to lower the pH in the colon.

10. **Goitrogenic foods** which if eaten in excess can affect your thyroid in a negatively. They are commonly known as Goitrogenic foods, which means they contain substances which can prevent your thyroid from getting its necessary amount of iodine. If eaten in excess, they interfere with the healthy function of your thyroid gland, tilting you in the direction of being even more hypothyroid, or making you susceptible to having a goiter, or enlargement of your thyroid. If you look closely at the word itself, you can see the root word is goiter (goitro-gen).

Bok choy

Broccoli

Brussels sprouts

Cabbage

Cauliflower

Garden kress

Kale

Kohlrabi

Mustard

Mustard greens

Radishes

Rutabagas

Soy

Soy milk

Soybean oil

Soy lecithin

Soy anything

Tempeh

Tofu

Turnips

Also included in the goitrogen category, even if mildly, are:

Bamboo shoots

Millet

Peaches

Peanuts

Pears

Pine nuts

Radishes

Spinach

Strawberries

Sweet potatoes

11. **Avoid Diet soda**- diet soda is a chemical cocktail made up of artificial sweeteners like aspartame, saccharin, and sucralose. Artificial sweeteners trigger insulin, which sends your body into fat storage mode and leads to weight gain. I go further into the insulin discussion later in the book. I want you to become aware of how sugar spikes affect your body weight.

12. **Avoid store brand Yogurt**- Conventional yogurt usually comes from milk produced by cows that are confined and unable to graze in open pasture. They're usually fed GMO grains, not grass. As the yogurt ferments, chemical defoamers are sometimes added. Then high doses of artificial sweeteners, sugar, or high fructose corn syrup are sometimes added too. That's not all: colors, preservatives, and gut-harmful carrageenan can be dumped in.

13. **Avoid High fructose corn syrup** - read labels, stay away from any products that contain this, it is 20x sweeter than sugar and our bodies don't recognize HFCS. What happens when our bodies doesn't recognize something? It turns it into fat. It also confuses your body &* doesn't let your brain know when your full!

Have you ever stopped to think what the underlying reason why you have hypothyroidism?

Many different underlying reasons can play a role. We do know that hypothyroidism is a chronic condition of an underactive thyroid and affects millions of Americans. Environmental chemicals and toxins, pesticides, BPA, thyroid endocrine disruptors, iodine imbalance, other medications, fluoride, overuse of soy products, cigarette smoking, and gluten intolerance. All of these play a very important role in your thyroid health. A nonprofit group called Beyond Pesticides warns that some 60 percent of pesticides used today have been shown to affect the thyroid gland's production of T3 and T4 hormones. Commercially available insecticides and fungicides have also been involved. Even dental x-rays have been linked to an increased risk of thyroid disorders.

Other causes:

Iodine deficiency

Hashimoto's Thyroiditis

Certain medications eg- lithium based mood stabilizers

Viral infection

Radiation therapy to the neck area

Radioactive iodine treatment

Thyroid surgery

Pituitary gland disorder

Hypothyroidism means what exactly?

Hypothyroidism means your thyroid is not making enough thyroid hormone. Your thyroid is a butterfly-shaped gland in the front of your throat. It makes the hormones that control the way your body uses energy. Basically, our thyroid hormone tells all the cells in our bodies how busy they should be. Our bodies will go into overdrive with too much thyroid hormone (hyperthyroidism) and our bodies slow down with too little thyroid hormone (hypothyroidism). The most common causes of hypothyroidism worldwide is dietary and environmental. The most common cause of hypothyroidism is dietary and environmental! What does that mean exactly? That means you need to be eat to cater to your thyroid and stop using all these harmful chemicals to clean your home with and put on your body! It's not hard. Yes, a little adjustment will be needed but isn't everything we do in life for the better of our health worth a little inconvenience until it becomes a habit?

Here are a list of symptoms that Hypothyroidism can cause:

- Dry skin and brittle nails
- Your fingertips becoming numb
- Feeling fatigued, weak, or depressed
- Constipation
- Memory problems or having trouble thinking clearly
- Heavy or irregular menstrual periods
- Joint or muscle pain
- Dry skin
- Hair loss
- Headaches
- Unexplained weight gain
- Thinning hair
- Clammy palms
- Difficulty swallowing
- Sensation of lump in throat
- Dry, itchy scalp
- Diminished sex drive
- Persistent cold sores, boils, or breakouts
- Elevated levels of LDL (the "bad" cholesterol)
- Heightened risk of heart disease
- Heart Palpitations
- Inability to lose weight

Inability to eat in the mornings

Tightness in throat; sore throat; horse sounding voice

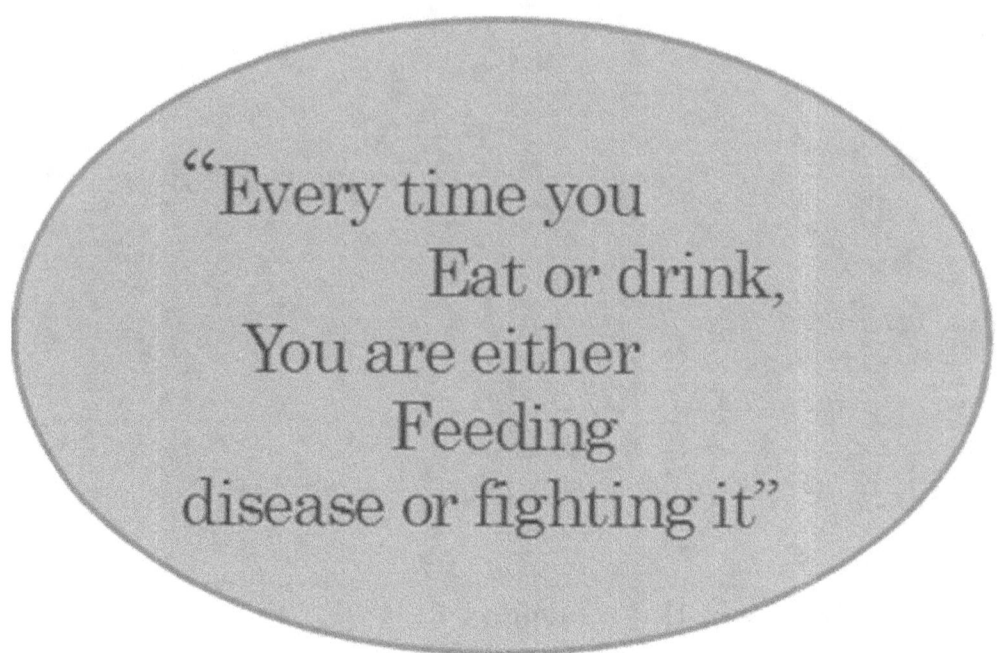

Breakfast

Start your morning out with a warm lemon water. Along with your thyroid medication. Wait 1 hour then drink your smoothie.

Hypothyroidism approved breakfast:

Hypothyroidism shake: You have 21 hypothyroidism approved shakes with vegan protein powder to pick from.

Lunch

Hypothyroidism approved lunch:

You have 21 delicious hypothyroidism approved salad in jar lunches to pick from. They are packed full of nutrients, healthy fats and proteins. Along with your lunch you should take your vitamins and probiotics. **Why take a probiotic?** Probiotic's can help restore our internal balance and will increase our vibrancy and overall health. It improved our digestive functions, improves our liver functions, improves resistance to allergies, improves energy, and improves the absorption of nutrients and help to eliminate bloating and heartburn.

Dinner

Hypothyroidism approved dinner:

You have 21 entrée-sized salads with healthy fats and quality proteins. Along with a warm cup of healthy bone broth.

After dinner take a short 10 minute walk or do some yoga stretches. A short walk or some yoga stretches will help your digestion, move along those bowl movements & reduce stress. Pamper yourself with an Epsom salt bath a few times during your reboot. 1 cup of Epsom salt, 1 cup of baking soda and 3 drops of lavender.

Bone broth goes well beyond its taste and warmth. There's a reason why it's called the magic elixir. Bone Broth boosts your collagen which makes Your Hair, Skin, and Nails Look Dead Sexy. One of the most vital nutrients for healing the gut is gelatin which bone broth is loaded with! The gelatin in bone broth acts like a spackle and heals the excess holes in the gut lining. Bone broth has glucosamine which protect your joints. The glycine in bone broth has been shown in several studies to help people sleep better and improve memory. Bone marrow from the bone broth can help strengthen your immune system. A Harvard study even showed that some people with auto-immune disorders experienced a relief of symptoms when drinking bone broth, with some achieving a complete remission. I also have a vegan gut healing broth recipe in this book.

After you have successfully rocked your 21 day reboot. You will need to continue your journey with more ultimate and amazing Hypothyroidism recipes. The single most important thing you can do is start eating The Hypothyroidism way. I've written 9 books in total. Please look for it in books store and online. If your book store doesn't carry it please request that it does. You need unprocessed recipes that will refuel-your-body, supercharge your metabolism, revitalize thyroid function, and help you continue to shed those excess pounds! Along with bonus recipes for nontoxic house hold cleaning ideas. It's not about being skinny, it's about gaining energy, vitality, and feeling good when you look in the mirror." I hope you become inspired.

Also, that's not all! If you are pressed for time and have no time in the kitchen?

All of my books are like having closely guarded secrets in the palm your hands! You never have to worry about what you're eating and they are all surprisingly simple!

Please check out my books online @ Amazon, Barnes n Noble or Books a Million.

Awareness has Magic: Creating a Healthy Hypothyroidism Mind, body and Spirit Home life

We must take a stand for our health. Your Thyroid hormones affect every organ in your body, every tissue and every single cell. You must start rebalancing the immune system by addressing the root cause of your hypothyroidism. Throughout this book, you will find useful, informative and easy to understand recipes for your entire essence. When I started writing this book, I wanted to introduce you to the idea of a cleaner less toxic world and for you to learn just how simply easy it is for you to start creating your own cleaning recipes throughout your home but this book has transformed into so much more than just a book full of all natural DIY recipes. This book will enlighten you and help you have a deeper understanding of not only why you should be more aware but how to be more aware.

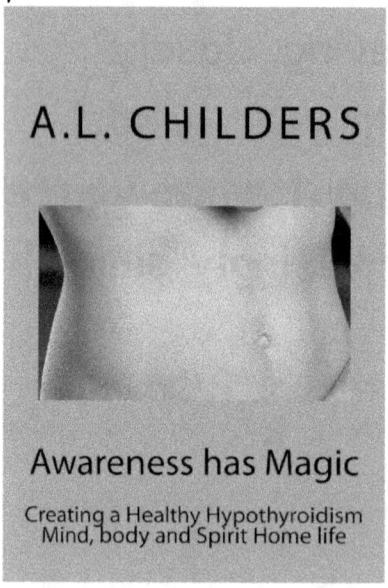

Holiday Hypothyroidism

Finally a Holiday cookbook that will have you sincerely appreciating all the hard work that I put into creating it. This cookbook not only has recipes that caters to your hypothyroidism but the recipes are extremely easy to prepare while still being delicious as they promote your health, help you begin to heal, and you're eating cleaner on top of it all. These recipes can be used year-round not only around the holidays and will be a great addition to your library. I hope you find this Holiday book a godsend to the particularly crazy holiday season. This book includes a good variety of recipes that I know you will find to be delicious, full of flavor, healthy and just perfect for your Thanksgiving and Christmas dinner table. From appetizers to main meals, side dishes and desserts these recipes are just wonderfully delicious. I am not kidding when I tell you that the recipe options in this book are endless and you won't be disappointed! You will be able to find that perfect recipe in this book that makes your taste buds soar, fits your dietary needs and has your family bragging on your cooking skills. They may even think you secretly took lessons from Gordon Ramsay or Julia Childs

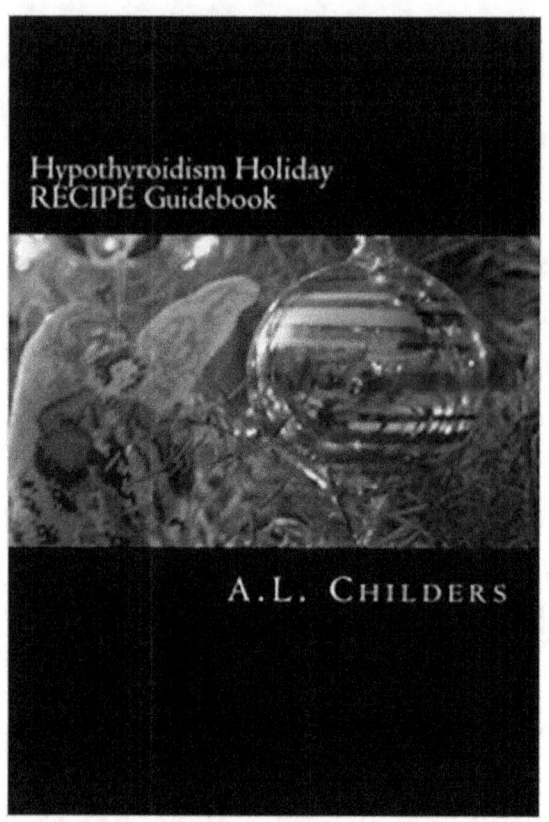

Secrets to my Hypothyroidism Success: A personal guide to Hypothyroidism freedom

I wish somebody had given me a step-by-step road-map back when I was first diagnosed with hypothyroidism. The solutions in this book has helped so many people. I've done my best to pull from all their expertise, as well as my own knowledge and clinical experience. I want to make it easy for you to find the answers quickly, all in the one place, because I'm all too familiar with that awful side effects of hypothyroidism. I certainly don't want you to have to spend years finding solutions, like I did. I also want you to understand that there isn't an easy "one pill" solution, but the "one pill" approach that our current medical system is using is NOT WORKING because the underlying cause for hypothyroidism is not being addressed. Knowledge is power, educate yourself and find the answer to your health care needs. Wisdom is a wonderful thing to seek. I hope this book will teach and encourage you to take leaps in your life to educate yourself for a happier & healthier life. You have to take ownership of your health

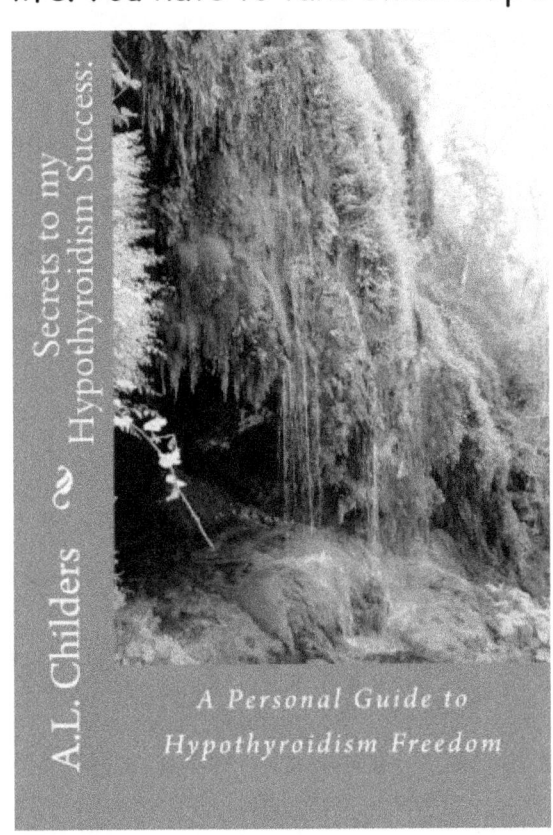

The Best Little Hypothyroidism Autumn Cookbook

I wanted to create a fall cookbook for those of us suffering from hypothyroidism that makes you feel as if you're inviting an old friend in for coffee. If you've been considering switching to a hypothyroidism diet, you may be wondering if you have to give up your favorite foods along with flavor. This is far from the truth. Switching to a hypothyroidism diet means that you are catering to heal your thyroid. You can still enjoy your favorite fall recipes following a hypothyroidism diet- you'll just need to learn what substitutions you will need to make to create wonderful fall hypothyroidism recipes. This is where this book that I've written for you comes into play. In this book, you will find a collection of many fall favorite recipes that you and your family are sure to love. If you've ever considered a hypothyroidism diet, this recipe book is a great starting resource.

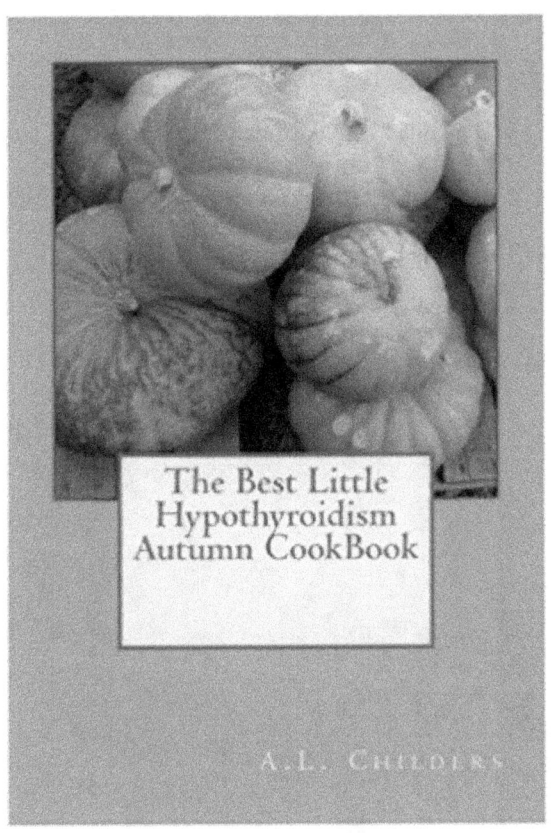

Hashimoto's crock-pot recipes: Added Bonus: How I put my Hashimoto's into remission

There's nothing like the aroma of a home-cooked dinner welcoming you at the door. No time to be in the kitchen? The wonderful thing about a crock pot is you have little prep time. You won't have to stand over a hot stove cooking your food and it's perfect for those hectic days. We all want that convenience! Do you need foods that promote thyroid health? You can start today healing your body from the inside out. Over 101 wholesome and nourishing Hashimoto's fighting recipes that will cater to your mind, body and soul. This helpful book will start to guide you in the right direction along with a step by step plan that is clear and doable.

It's not about being skinny, it's about energy, vitality & feeling good when you look in the mirror.

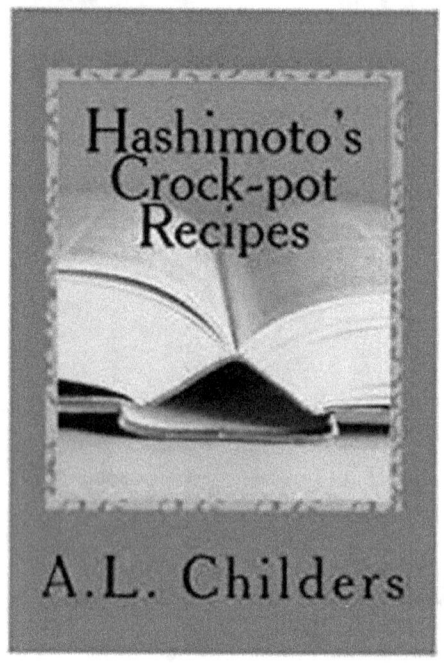

A Survivors Cookbook Guide to Kicking Hypothyroidism's booty.

Do you need foods that promote your thyroid health? Let's heal your body from the inside out. We've all heard that our gut is called the "second-brain". Given how closely the two interact with each other one thing you may not realize is your emotions and weight gain can start in the gut. Your gut and digestion can also cause you to hold onto that excess weight and just feel lousy. I've included 101 hypothyroidism fighting recipes that cook themselves. Our main concern is kicking hypothyroidism's booty. I hope this book inspires you to use your slow cooker more often and create your own new recipes. Let's together shed those extra pounds, regain your self-confidence and vitality back into your life.

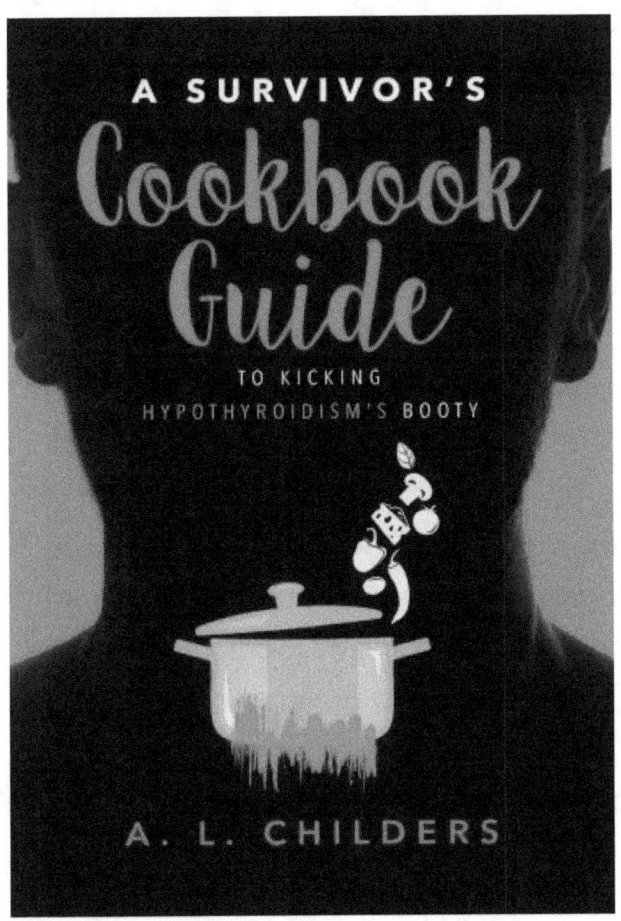

Hypothyroidism: The beginners Guide

This book thanks everyone suffering from hypothyroidism and looking for answers. Hypothyroidism is the kind of disease that carries a bit of mystery with it. This book is not for readers looking for quick answers. There is not one size fits all. You have to be in charge of your health. I didn't write this book to sell you any "snake oil" in a bottle. I've written this book to be an eye opener for you and to share with you what I have learned on my journey. The solutions in this book has helped so many people. There are many incredible holistic practitioners, authors and researchers with experience and expertise in this area. I've done my best to pull from all their expertise, as well as my own knowledge and clinical experience. I want to make it easy for you to find the answers quickly, all in the one place, because I'm all too familiar with that awful side effects of hypothyroidism. I certainly don't want you to have to spend years finding solutions, like I did. I also what you to understand that there isn't an easy "one pill" solution, but the "one pill" approach that our current medical system is using is NOT WORKING because the underlying cause for hypothyroidism is not being addressed. Get ready to go on a journey of discovery where you are going to learn how everything ties into one. A lack of knowledge is a lack of power.

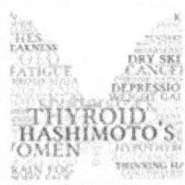

Hypothyroidism: The Beginners Guide

How to Stop Surviving and Start Thriving

A.L Childers

Kicking Hypothyroidism's booty, The Slow Cooker way: 101 Slow Cooker recipes!

I wanted to create a user-friendly handbook to help anyone affected by this disorder. I've seen many doctors over the years and none offered me ideas on diet change. I've included recipes, ideas on solutions for a healthier home, what you should be eating and shouldn't, how to shed those extra pounds, regain your self-confidence and vitality back into your life. I want you to feel strong, sexy, and beautiful. This is my heartfelt guide to you. Together, once again, you can start to gain that wonderful life that you deserve. I am a student in this thing called life. I want to be remembered as a pioneer who thought, imagined, and inspired. What we feel at times is the impossible or unthinkable. Life is a wonderful journey.

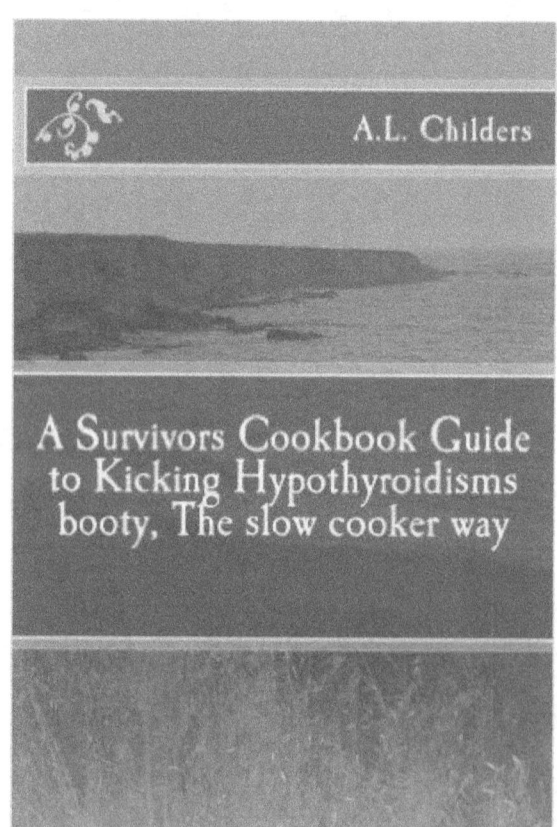

Beauty Tip!

Mediating and looking more Toned

Any time you change your diet from unhealthy to a healthier way of eating you should always exercise to help release toxins that have been sitting in your body from years of improper digestion, preservatives from our foods , poisons in our skin care products, pollutions, house hold chemicals , stress and along with other things. Sweating when you exercise is one way to cleanse your body and help release those toxins that has built up in your body. Yoga is wonderful to help tone, slows your mind process down and relieves stress. A nice steamed sauna is excellent to help pull out those toxins too. My local YMCA has a steam sauna room and I use it frequently. Our body is a wonderful, fantastic thing. It has its own eliminative organs which include the lungs, liver kidneys, colon, and your skin. Sometimes you will notice detoxing changes in the way of acne, rashes, colds and flu. When this happens what do we normally do? Take medications to fix it or put medications on it. Why not fix the root of the issue instead of covering up the issue. Your body is trying to tell you it's overloaded with toxicity. What you do? You can start eating right. Be mindful of what you put in your mouth. Before you take that next bite ask yourself: How is this feeding my body with nutrients? Remember, with every bite of food you consume your either fighting disease or feeding disease. Once you start on your journey. You might feel a bit more bloated, a headache, even a skin rash, aches and pains, soreness and moodiness. Don't be alarmed and this is only temporary. All those years of toxic build up in your body is making its way out of your body! Stay strong by the end of your 21 day reboot you will feel and look incredible and your body will be thanking you. So will those jeans too!

Has your body turned into a fat magnet?

Hypothyroidism is very common and it's estimated that 27 million Americans have some kind of thyroid imbalance. That butterfly-shaped gland that is located in the front of your neck, just below your Adam's apple produces thyroid hormone. These hormones helps to control the rate at which your body burns calories (as well as your heart rate, body temperature, digestion, fertility, mood, and a host of other functions). When your thyroid isn't working properly the hormones become imbalanced and this chemical reaction will throw off your entire body. Do you wonder why you feel sluggish, no energy and you are piling on the pounds no matter how healthy you're eating.

When you hear the word hormonal imbalance for some reason we think of menopause in women. This can't be further from the truth. If you have to much of the hormone estrogen being produced it creates more body fat and within that body fat it contains an enzyme that converts adrenal steroids into believing it needs to create more body fat . It's an ugly cycle where your body fat will continue to produce more estrogen and in return continue to create more body fat. This is where your body becomes confused and is unable to effectively use body fat as energy so it starts to get stored. Your hormonal imbalance also creates changes in your body's blood sugar levels where it will releases insulin more often.

Signs & Symptoms of Hormonal Imbalances

Some of the most common signs and symptoms of hormone imbalances include:

- Infertility and irregular periods
- Weight gain or weight loss (that's unexplained and not due to intentional changes in your diet)
- Depression and anxiety
- Fatigue
- Insomnia
- Low libido
- Changes in appetite
- Digestive issues
- Hair loss and hair thinning

Hormonal imbalances just don't happen overnight. There are many contributing life factors from leaky gut syndrome, genetics, and exposure to toxins in the environment, endocrine disrupting body lotions and potions, stress, medical history, body inflammation, being overweight, lack of sleep, pesticides being sprayed on our foods.

You're not going to be able to heal your adrenals, balance your hormones, and get your thyroid levels into a normal range overnight. It will be a process just like it took a process to get you here.

Steps to Balancing Your Hormones Naturally

1. Meditation

Start your day off with meditation and a grateful heart. There are many people who weren't able to wake up and live another day. I can't even begin to express the importance of the power of meditation has over the body. It's been proven to lower your lower the levels of cortisol which is also known as the stress hormone. I like to start my day off listening to mediation music to clear my head while I am have my legs up the wall yoga pose.

Legs up the wall pose will not only help with your thyroid functions but it also relieves back pain, helps with insomnia, improves posture, helps with anxiety, naturally adjusts your spine, improves your digestion and it starts a lymphatic circulation. Your lymphatic system doesn't have a pump and relies on our movements and gravity to circulate lymph fluid where the toxins in this fluid can be eliminated from your body. If we sit all day the lymph fluid becomes stagnant and start to collect toxins. By simply reversing the flow of gravity in your legs, you begin to circulate the lymphatic fluid and encourage the body to start the elimination of toxins. Dry brushing also will simulate the lymphatic system and improve skin tone.

2. Keeping your blood sugar in check

Metabolic Syndrome is real and if your body has been on a blood sugar roller coaster is highly likely that you have developed this disorder. High cortisol levels can also interfere with how the body regulates the use of blood sugar.

You need to start eating foods that help manage blood sugar levels and are good for your thyroid like: wild fish such as salmon, free-range eggs, grass-fed beef or lamb, raw dairy products (including yogurt, kefir or raw cheeses), and pasture-raised poultry. Sea vegetables: Kelp, nori, kombu, dulse, arame, wakame, hijiki. Seafood: Haddock, clams, salmon, shrimp, oysters, sardines.garlic, asparagus, mushrooms, summer squash, sesame seeds, lima beans, sunflower seeds, Brazil nuts, ginger root, cinnamon, white beans, pumpkin seeds, blackstrap molasses, kiwifruit, parsley, peppers (chili, Bell, sweet), Start consuming Essential fatty acids are the building blocks for our hormones like fatty fish and shellfish, flaxseed and flaxseed oil, hemp seed, olive oil, chia seeds, pumpkin seeds, sunflower seeds, leafy vegetables, and walnuts. Healthy fats like: virgin coconut oil, MCT oil, extra virgin olive oil, nuts and seeds (like almonds, chia, hemp and flax), and avocado. Coconut oil, ghee and grass-fed butters. Adding more High-fiber foods like: fresh veggies, whole pieces of fruit (not juice), sprouted beans or peas, quinoa, artichokes, green leafy vegetables, chia seeds, flaxseeds, apples, pumpkin seeds, almonds, avocado and sweet potatoes. Don't be afraid to eat eggs! Due to the selenium content, Egg yolks are nature's thyroid support supplement. 40% of the selenium is found in the white and 60% are found in the yolk. Egg yolks also has REAL vitamin A, Vitamin D which is a fat-soluble vitamin and we certainly don't get enough of that and the good cholesterol in egg yolks helps also to balance hormones. Try to stick with non-starchy vegetables such as cooked broccoli, cucumbers, and carrots. Non-starchy vegetables can also help prevent surges in blood sugar levels while providing essential nutrients. Also Bragg's apple cider vinegar has been proven to improve fasting blood sugar levels and insulin sensitivity. All you need to consume is 2ounces per day

3. **Avoid Processed foods**

Anything that has been made in a lab and by man just avoid. It is vital that you start to eat a diet full of nutrient-dense foods that your body will be able to easily digest, absorb, and your body can use as fuel.

4. Fix your gut

Probiotics can help to begin repairing the lining in your gut. This also aids in helping to balance your hormones. if someone has leaky gut syndrome it allows undigested food particles to leak through your gut into your bloodstream and in return creates disease-causing inflammation that will have an impact on your body — especially your thyroid glands where they are very susceptible to inflammation.

5. Sleep

A lack of long term sleep can raise cortisol levels. You should aim for 7-8 hours of sleep every night.

6. Taking the right supplements

Natural vs. Synthetic Vitamins - What's the Big Difference?

Supplementing your body with the nutrients it that it is lacking is very important step in balancing hormones. Stress can lead to a deficiency in B vitamins, magnesium, zinc, vitamin C and chromium. Selenium and iodine are other key components in the production and conversion of thyroid hormones so if you are lacking these vital nutrients it will be harder for your thyroid to work as it needed.

Vitamins are little organic molecules we need, but we can't make them or at least we have a hard time making them ourselves. We must rely on our food to keep us stocked with these essential nutrients, but our food is getting less and less nutritious. Fields are depleted by overuse. Pesticides limit the action of beneficial microbes in the soil that help plants draw in nutrients. Fertilizers focus on certain key chemicals and don't take into account all the trace minerals, organic components, or beneficial microbes that go into good nutrition. And genetically modified foods have made their way into our food supply when we don't know how they may affect us in the long term.

We refine and process our food so it lasts longer, is more convenient, tastes better, and is even made to be more addictive. We strip out and destroy vital nutrients as we process them. Much of the food we find in grocery stores outside the produce section barely resembles what humanity has been eating for thousands of years. There's no wonder we have so many auto-immune disorders, food allergies, and growing epidemics of obesity. Our bodies don't know what we're ingesting, they aren't finding the nutrients they need, and they're begging for us to eat more and more so we might manage to give ourselves what we're missing.

We all know we need a steady supply of vitamins and minerals so our bodies can function properly. Scientists, doctors, and food companies agree too, so they create cheap vitamins in labs, fortify our foods and beverages with them, and dump them into multivitamins. The problem is these synthetic vitamins are not what our bodies are looking for either. I've found that all Garden Of Life products are fantastic. You should also get your doctor to perform a routine blood work to see what your body is lacking.

7. Detox your lifestyle

We are creating a toxic shit storm within our very own bodies. I'm not speaking from a place of Prejudice or judgement because what you do with your life is entirely your call. The real reality is we are damaging our DNA and we are changing our genetic makeup for future generations. These chemicals in our food, beverages, vaccines and pharmaceuticals create a breeding ground for sickness. Have you heard of gene mutation? It's when the cells are changed by chemicals they are either damaged, lost or copied. These processed foods that are full of man-made chemicals, fluoridated municipal tap water, genetically modified foods, Artificial sweeteners,

Vaccines and the yearly flu shot – often contain mercury, aluminum, formaldehyde and MSG, Pharmaceutical medications and a lot of the Pharmaceutical medications are loaded with fluoride, OTC (over-the-counter) medications for colds, allergies, headaches and fever – often contain heavy metal toxins, artificial sweeteners and toxic industrial-based food dyes. All of this is what is keeping us sick and these corporations rich.

Did you know that most of these products we use every day contain toxic chemicals and has been linked to women's health issues? They are hidden endocrine disruptors and are very tricky chemicals that play havoc on our bodies. "We are all routinely exposed to endocrine disruptors, and this has the potential to significantly harming our health. In my book, Awareness has Magic, I have a ton of all natural nontoxic recipes.

8. Essential oils

Essential oils are more than a plant based therapy. They represent a way of life that empowers people to regain control of their health. The internet if filled with stories of how people's lives have been changed by essential oils. Some of these testimonials will touch your heart and others will inspire you to revisit the products that you use and your approach to your health care. When I started using essentials oils it changed my life in a way that was unprecedented. For the 1st time ever, I am here to talk about my life in this no judgment zone. I am talking from a safe place I learned how to address health my concerns, where I enhanced my performance and I found some tools that pointed me to a new way of life. They have the ability to lower cortisol levels, promote a calming effects on the body, and boost thyroid hormone production. Rosemary, peppermint, frankincense, myrrh, and lavender are excellent. Many others like Clary sage, geranium, ylang ylang, and lavender have the ability to restore balance in the female reproductive system, normalizing estrogen and testosterone levels. Copaiba is an essential oil that helps treat inflammation associated with thyroid problems. With rich amount of caryophyllene, it strengthens the body's natural reaction to irritation and injuries.

9. Try Adaptogen Herbs

Adaptogen herbs are in a unique class of healing plants that promote hormone balance and help to protect the body from a wide variety of diseases, including those caused by excess stress. They also boost your immune functions. Research shows that various adapotogens — such as ashwagandha, medicinal mushrooms, rhodiola and holy basil Studies show that holy basil can helps to regulate cortisol level, protect your organs and tissues against chemical stress from pollutants and heavy metals, which are other factors that can lead to hormone imbalance. — The unique healing herbs can—

- Improve thyroid function
- Lower cholesterol naturally
- Reduce anxiety and depression
- Reduce brain cell degeneration
- Stabilize blood sugar and insulin levels
- Support adrenal gland functions

10. Avoid all Caffeine

Nothing like that waking up to the smell of coffee. Its gets the juices flowing with that very 1st sip. Its offer you an energetic boost and mental clarity on a feeling that life can go on.

The thyroid gland is such a very important part of the body's regulatory mechanisms; thyroid problems can affect everything in the body from our temperature to appetite to the pulse. Caffeine, a stimulant found in coffee, can affect the thyroid in a number of ways and has an effect on your central nervous system, your digestive tract, and your metabolism.

According to the recent article, in new study from the journal Thyroid people who consume coffee at the time of taking their thyroid medication, we see a 25-57% drop in T4, one of the thyroid hormones, compared to non-coffee drinkers. This adverse effect persists for up to one hour.

Researchers have also found that for patients taking levothyroxine tablets, absorption is affected by drinking coffee and espresso within an hour of taking the thyroid drugs.

According to "Coffee and Health," by Gerard Debry, in experiments on rats, very high doses of caffeine caused the thyroid gland to enlarge, but at doses of about 300 mg, caffeine in humans did not change levels of thyroid hormones.

What about the benefits? Yes, there are many reliable studies that say coffee is full of antioxidants and polyphenols. However, these same antioxidants and polyphenols can also be found abundantly in many fruits and vegetables.

There are many other reliable studies that show coffee can play a role in the prevention of cancer, diabetes, depression, cirrhosis of the liver, gallstones, etc.

Many coffee drinkers report feeling good for the first two hours (mainly due to a dopamine spike).

(If you just can't give up that morning cup of Joe recommendations by researchers are clear: wait at least sixty minutes after taking levothyroxine before drinking coffee.)

10-1. Increases blood sugar levels

According to this study, caffeine increases blood sugar levels. This is especially dangerous for people with hypoglycemia (or low sugar levels) who feel jittery, shaky, moody and unfocused when hungry. Blood sugar fluctuations cause cortisol spikes, which not only exhaust the adrenals, but also deregulate the immune system. This is highly undesirable for those of us with adrenal fatigue, Hashimoto's or Graves' disease. Such cortisol spikes are also highly inflammatory.

10-2. Creates sugar and carbohydrate cravings

As the result of the above, when our blood sugar levels come down, we need an emergency fix to bring them back up. This is why people who drink coffee at breakfast or indulge in sugary and processed breakfasts crave carbs and sugar by 11am or later in the day.

10-3. Contributes to acid reflux and damages gut lining

Coffee stimulates the release of gastrin, the main gastric hormone, which speeds up intestinal transit time. Coffee can also stimulate the release of bile (which is why some people run to the bathroom soon after drinking coffee) and digestive enzymes.

In a person with a healthy digestion, this is not a big deal. However, for people with autoimmune conditions, compromised digestion (such as IBS, or "leaky gut"), this can cause further digestive damage to the intestinal lining.

10-4. **Exhausts the adrenals**

Coffee stimulates the adrenals to release more cortisol, our stress hormone; this is partly why we experience a wonderful but temporary and unsustainable burst of energy.

What many of us don't realize is that our tired adrenals are often the cause of unexplained weight gain, sleeping problems, feeling emotionally fragile, depression and fatigue. Drinking coffee while experiencing adrenal fatigue is only adding fuel to the fire.

10-5. **Worsens PMS and lumpy breasts**

It's well-established that coffee contributes to estrogen dominance (source), which can mean one of two things: we either have too much estrogen in relation to progesterone, or we have an imbalance in the estrogen metabolites (some are protective and some are dangerous).

PMS, lumpy breasts, heavy periods, cellulite and even breast cancer (which is an estrogenic cancer) can be symptoms of estrogen dominance.

10-6. Gluten-cross reactive food

50% of people with gluten sensitivities also experience cross reactivity with other foods, including casein in milk products, corn, coffee, and almost all grains, because their protein structures are similar. Cyrex Labs provides a test for gluten cross-reactive foods.

Many people report having a similar reaction to coffee as they do to gluten.

10-7. Impacts the conversion of T4 to T3 thyroid hormones

Coffee impacts the absorption of levothyroxine (the synthetic thyroid hormone); this is why thyroid patients need to take their hormone replacement pill at least an hour before drinking coffee.

The indirect but important point is that coffee contributes to estrogen dominance, cited above, and estrogen dominance inhibits T4 to T3 conversion.

10-8. Can cause miscarriages

This study showed that women who drink coffee during their pregnancy are at a higher risk of miscarriage.

10-9. is highly inflammatory

Any functional or integrative doctor would say the majority of modern diseases are caused by inflammation – a smoldering and invisible fire found on a cellular level.

This study found that caffeine is a significant contributor to oxidative stress and inflammation in the body. Chronic body pains and aches, fatigue, skin problems, diabetes and autoimmune conditions are just some of the conditions related to inflammation.

10-10. Can contribute to and even cause osteoporosis

It is well-known that coffee changes our body pH to a lower, and thus more acidic, level. A low pH (which means a more acidic body) can contribute to osteoporosis.

This study has confirmed that habitual coffee drinking among postmenopausal women was the leading cause of osteoporosis.

10-11. Can cause insomnia and poor sleep

This study showed that 400mg of "caffeine taken 6 hours before bedtime has important disruptive [sleep] effects."

This rich creamy and lightly sweet beverage is something you're sure to enjoy!

Turmeric Tea Recipe

Total Time: 5 minutes

Serves: 2

Ingredients:

1 cup coconut milk

1 cup water

1 tbsp. ghee

1 tbsp. honey

1 tsp Turmeric (powder or grated root)

Directions:

Pour coconut milk and water into the saucepan and warm for 2 minutes

Add in butter, raw honey and turmeric powder for another 2 minutes

Stir and pour into glasses.

You have to exercise caution when combining it with medications or supplements taken to slow down blood clotting. Turmeric supplements must be stopped two weeks prior to a surgery.

11. Infrared Sauna Therapy

Infrared saunas help your body balance hormones by increasing your metabolic rate, helps to release a toxins, including heavy metals like mercury and lead, and environmental chemicals, it also assists in weight loss by helping you burn up to 600 calories in a single sauna session and is comparable are to a 6 to 9 mile run. It Increases your circulation, and helps to purify your skin.

12. Magnesium Oil

Mineral balance goes hand-and-hand with hormone balance.

Calming Magnesium Body Butter

My homemade magnesium body butter will help replace the magnesium that our bodies need to thrive to survive. I always try to apply a little to my feet and shoulders before bed. This helps me relax and also get a fantastic night's sleep. It's pretty easy to make and the benefits are overwhelming. Magnesium deficiency is very common and it mimics other common symptoms and many other conditions like, being tired and felling run down, not sleeping well, getting headaches, gut issues, and even feeling stressed and anxious.

Here is a list of things that can lower our magnesium levels:

Too much caffeine

Processed food and Sugar

Too much stress

Poor sleep habits

Calming Magnesium Body Butter

1/2 cup cocoa butter

1/2 cup of coconut oil and melt

1/4 cup magnesium oil

Add 10 drops of lavender essential oil

Add 10 drops cedar wood essential oil

Add 10 drops frankincense essential oil

Place a heat-safe glass measuring cup/bowl inside a pot that has 1-2 inches of simmering water over medium heat. Add the cocoa butter & Melt it in your double boiler until it's completely melted.

Remove the cocoa butter from heat, and add 1/2 cup extra virgin coconut oil to the melted cocoa butter and stir until completely the coconut oil has melted. Next add 1/4 cup magnesium oil to the mixture and combine. Place the mixture in the refrigerator to cool for about 30-60 minutes (until it is cooled completely). After the mixture has completely cooled and became a solid. Use a hand mixer or stand mixer to whip it. Start on low and increase speed slowly. Whip for about 3-5 minutes. Next add the 10 drops each of lavender essential oil, the 10 drops of cedar wood essential oil, and the 10 drops of frankincense essential oil. Scrape down the sides of the bowl and continue whipping for another 5 minutes or so, until the magnesium body butter is light and fluffy. The color of the magnesium body butter will change from yellow to a pale ivory and almost white color. Lastly put the magnesium body butter into mason jars and seal tightly with a lid. Make sure to label and date the top of the lid. This recipe makes enough for two 4 oz. glass jars.

13. **Avoid SOY!**

Soy not only disrupts hormones by mimicking estrogen in your body but it also causes inflammation, contributes to leaky gut syndrome and most likely has been genetically modified (GMO). Start reading your labels. You will be surprised how companies will sneak in soy.

Brilliant marketing campaigns have lead you to believe that soy products are healthy but in fact it's completely the opposite. Soy products are not healthy foods. Eating soy frequently can potentially lead to numerous other health issues.

For centuries, Asian people have been consuming fermented soy products such as natto, tempeh, and soy sauce, and enjoying the health benefits. Fermented soy does not wreak havoc on your body like unfermented soy products do.

The issue with soy is most soy today contains something called phytoestrogens, and these phytoestrogens are estrogen mimickers in the body. And so, if you're a male consuming extra estrogen, it's going to give you more feminine characteristics.

If you're a woman consuming foods that increase estrogen levels, it's going to increase your risk of breast cancer, cervical cancer, PCOS (polycystic ovary syndrome) and other hormone imbalance-related disorders.

Many have felt as if they needed a diary substitute since they couldn't tolerate dairy. Actually your body was doing you an even bigger favor.

For starters, some chemicals such as isoflavones, found in soy products like soy milk or edamame, can intercept your thyroid's ability to make hormones if you're not getting enough iodine.

Soybeans are one of the crops that are being genetically modified. Since 1997 GMO soybeans are being used in an increasing number of products.

Dr. Kaayla Daniel, author of **The Whole Soy Story**, points out thousands of studies linking soy to malnutrition, digestive distress, immune-system breakdown, thyroid dysfunction, cognitive decline, reproductive disorders and infertility—even cancer and heart disease. Here is just a sampling of the health effects that have been linked to soy consumption:

Breast cancer

Brain damage

Infant abnormalities

Thyroid disorders

Kidney stones

Immune system impairment

Severe, potentially fatal food allergies

Impaired fertility

Danger during pregnancy and nursing

Final thoughts on Soy: Soy is terrible – contains trypsin inhibitors, is a source of xenoestrogens, even if it's organic, and if it's GMO, it also comes with a lot of glyphosate and other pesticide residues. Avoid it like the black plague.

14. Invest in a water filter

The water that comes from your sink probably contains chlorine or fluoride (or both)—which can also disrupt the thyroid by interfering with its ability to absorb iodine properly that it needs to produce hormones. I use a Berkey Water Tank.

15. Start making your own household cleaning supplies and body lotions

It's not enough to be aware of all the outdoor chemicals that we are exposed to everyday but inside our homes we can have more power and control. We are a walking human chemical experiment for companies and they don't care about our health just lining their pockets with money. As humans, we need to open up our eyes and use a little common sense. We can be more aware about using chemical cleaners, paints, glues, body lotions, toothpastes, underarm deodorants, hair products and pesticides. Instead use products that don't pollute our very own bodies. We must read labels, make our own products and do our own research. I can't stress this enough. We must take a stand for our health. Stop using commercial products that are laced with unknown and harmful body damaging products. Your Thyroid hormones affect every organ in your body, every tissue and every single cell.

16. Drink plenty of water!

Drinking Water will help your body maintain the Balance of Bodily Fluids. Your body is made up of 60% water. The liquid helps your bodily fluids include digestion, absorption, circulation, creation of saliva, transportation of nutrients, and control of body's temperature. Try to think of water as a necessary nutrient to keep your body working. If your Cells don't maintain enough fluids and electrolytes it can result in muscle fatigue.

17. Food allergies

If you allergic to certain foods it is will involve you're the immune system. You know that your immune system controls how your body defends itself. For example if you have a food allergy to cow's milk, your immune system will see cow's milk as an invader. In return your immune system overreacts by producing antibodies called Immunoglobulin E (IgE). These antibodies travel to cells that release chemicals, causing an allergic reaction to start fighting for your body. Being tested for food allergies seems to be easiest way to check to see if you have any food allergies so you can start avoiding these foods and help your immune system become strong again.

16. Exercise

We all know that regular exercise is an important part of your overall health. Exercise burns calories to prevent weight gain and helps speed up your metabolism. It is also a releases endorphins to give you those mood-enhancing chemicals. What if I told you that exercise can cause adrenal crashes due to your already high cortisol issues? You could be stressing your thyroid out even more and not even realizing it. Are you exercising but not getting any results? Are you still gaining weight, feeling constantly fatigued, irritable and moody and often battling some other sort of sickness? You could be actually stressing your body more out by over-exercising.

The magic word here is cortisol.

Cortisol, a steroid hormone produced by the adrenal gland. It is released in response to stress. When you are stressed, your body releases certain "fight-or-flight" stress hormones that are produced in the adrenal glands: cortisol, norepinephrine and epinephrine. Staying stressed raises your cortisol levels and your body actually resists weight loss. Your body thinks times are hard and you might starve, so it hoards the fat you eat or what you have presently on your body. Cortisol will grab fat from your butt and hips, and move it to your abdomen which has more cortisol receptors. Hello there Mrs. Muffin Top!

Today most of us are in a chronic stress state. However, our body don't know the difference between car troubles, relationship issues, debt, work pressure and truly life-threatening stress. This is why our body still ready to defend and reacts exactly the same as it always has done.

Over-exercising can:

    Deplete hormones necessary for the functioning of the body

- Cause gradual bone loss
- Increase injuries
- Cause cramping of muscles
- Add to inflammation
- Increase healing time
- Affect cardiac function
- Affect blood flow
- Decrease the ability of muscles to use fatty acids as a source of energy
- Reduce endurance

My suggestion is to start off taking it easy. **Yoga, Pilates, walking, light weight lifting and swimming** are all great workouts for people with hypothyroidism.

Somethings you will see repeated in my book, perhaps many times over. I would think that should be a light bulb moment to take a better look at your life if you are still unable to heal. Start incorporating these suggestions in your life. One step, one day at a time and with each new day brings new opportunities.

Here are a few things you can start to incorporate into your life:

16-1. Limit your caffeine to 200 milligrams a day. (This is equal to about one 12 oz cup of coffee) Better yet, avoid all caffeine and start consuming Matcha tea, herbal teas and detox yourself from caffeine completely.

16-2. Start eating simple carbs, avoid processed foods, more anti-inflammatory foods, foods that are low on the G.I. Scale so you can avoid insulin spikes, refined grains (gluten) , and always get plenty of high-quality protein, healthy fats and great vegetables.

16-3. Its okay to say NO! Take time to relax, take a nap, distress and recuperate. Spend a day or two in your jammies relaxing. You deserve to have reboot time.

16-4. Start building your endurance back slowly. Take it easy. Start out with light weights and work your way to heavier ones. Start out with a 15 minute walk or a 15 minutes swim. You can do this many times in a day.

16-5. Get a heart rate monitor and use it. Know your heart rate comfort zone.

16-6. Listen to your body. How do you feel the next day? Do you need an extra day to recover?

16-7. Set realistic goals, one step at a time and don't get discouraged.

16-8. Remember Low-impact aerobics workouts. Something to get your heart rate up and your lungs going without putting too much pressure on your joints, which is important because joint pain is another common hypothyroidism symptom.

16-9. Strength training is good. Strength training builds muscle mass, and muscle burns more calories than fat, even when you're at rest.

16-10. Get some sleep!

Just think how great it's going to feel when you are as healthy on the inside as you look on the outside! The ultimate goal isn't to look fit but to be fit.

Did You Know That Your Body Has its Very Own Personal Food Code? 6 Tips

There is so much information overload that most women are confused as to where to start to begin creating a healthy lifestyle balance. Perhaps one of the biggest misconceptions is the ambivalence of it all. We all get super busy in this thing called life. Sometimes we lose a little piece of ourselves traveling back in fourth.

Although this book is a 21 day reboot with healthy-easy-to-do recipes. You will still need to find your personal food code eventually.

How many times this week have you said to yourself, "If my life wasn't so busy, I would be able to start exercising" or" Why did I eat that extra cookie?" or" its 3a.m., why can't I sleep?!" Or" Why am I so exhausted?"

Frankly, life is one big tug a war between feeling completely insane to the creativity at it all.

Why do we allow ourselves to become Stressed Out, Overwhelmed, and Totally Exhausted and continue to carry around those extra ungodly pounds that we dreadfully despise? After 5 years of carrying that excess weight, I am here to tell you, from one female to another, you can't technically call it baby weight gain any longer.

Have you ever wondered why people respond differently to losing weight?

In the last fifty years what has changed in our society? We have the same predisposition genetics as our grandparents. We are unique and come in all different shapes, sizes, race, religions and greed.

We can't blame is all on genetics being unhealthy solely on the DNA that was passed down to us. Everyone's genetic makeup is different. It's like your fingerprints.

In school, I was always that girl who was tall, skinny, freckled faced, wavy blonde hair with a flat chest and a flat butt. I remember being plagued at school for being too skinny. Having no shape. Tormented about my freckles. While other school mates were well endowed with large boobs, hippy hips and a nice rounder booty. Our metabolisms certainly dictate how we use energy and our genetics can dictate how we are shaped but what has started to interests me more-so lately is why we store fat on certain areas of our bodies when others don't.

These questions have confused and frustrated people and health care practitioners for decades. But why is it so confusing? One thing we have learned is each of us are unique and have our very own biochemistry that sets us apart from everyone else. Although we might share the same common traits and perhaps the same overlapping metabolic tendencies. We can't continue to say that one-size-fits-all when it comes to our very own unique body chemistry. There are over 7 billion people on this planet and we come in all different shapes, colors and sizes. With this being said wouldn't you think the one-size-fits-all- approach to losing weight wouldn't work since we are we are all unique. With this all being said wouldn't you think that we all have our very own personal food code too?

Finding Your Food Code

Finding your food code won't be as easy as it sounds. Quite frankly you will have to put some elbow grease into this but it's not unattainable. How we live from day to day is completely different on every spectrum across the board. One thing I do know for-sure is that every single day no matter who we are or where we live our bodies are bombarded with a toxic burden of chemicals, we are not feeding our bodies the proper nutrients, we are nutritional deficient, and some of us have little to no activity & these are some of the reasons why our bodies are becoming stagnant and increasingly polluted. It would be silly to take Motrin for a pebble stuck in your shoe when all you had to do was pluck it out. So why not on this journey go ahead, do some research and start addressing the issues at hand.

We are creating a perfect storm within our bodies. The less nutrients we consume, more toxins we add, create this world win of health issues. It's sad that our western diet is made up of red meats, vegetable oils, white flour and sugar. Who would have thought that something so simple as eating has become so complicated? Food does matter. It talks to your DNA. Food can change your DNA!

The foods you eat have a major impact your life — It affects your gut health and along with increasing or decreasing the inflammation in your body. Unfortunately, our western world diet are full of foods that have a bad impact on both your gut and your inflammation. If it was made in a lab, avoid it. Do a little research and you will find that our western diet that is made up of processed, fake foods, chemicals, sugar and corn oils are all highly flaming the fan of your inflammation.

We have a shortage of nutrients in our food system. The most common foods that you load up your grocery cart with are loaded with bad carbs, fillers, preservatives, additives, flavorings, and chemicals. Your body doesn't have any idea what do to with all this fake food. We are creating a weaker human race, inflammation and pain along with the possibility of welcoming other diseases and disorders. Your diet and lifestyle choices is what has caused any health issues that you may have unless you were born with a health issue then you can look at your parents diet , surroundings and lifestyle choices. It can go back generations. The only way to get back our health and vitality is to look at the root of it all.

You can change and control your life.

Think about what you're putting in your body. Either you're fighting disease or feeding disease. You must get a concept of nutrient density. Gluten, dairy and soy products create inflammation in the digestive tract. In ancient times grains were prepared by soaking, sprouting and fermenting but that tradition in making them been long forgotten with our fast-paced culture.

Let's talk more about store bought bread:

The bread you're buying at the store really isn't real bread you're buying. The white bread in the grocery is not the bread that our ancestors use to eat. 65% of the foods we eat are made from grains that are grown in a field such as grain bread, whiskey pasta and beer just to name a few. Wheat is made up of 3 parts the bran, the germ and the starchy endosperm.

The way the grain is processed has a huge impact not only on the way it taste and how healthy it is for you. Our ancestors used every part of the grain when they made their bread. White bread on the store shelves is made by a industrial process that strips out the wheat into all-purpose flour and in most cases if you read the back of the labels you will see chemicals additives added. These chemical additives is what gives white bread a longer shelve life.

White bread is also only made from the starchy endosperm which your body turns into pure sugar.

If you have inflammation in the digestive system undigested proteins leak into the blood stream creating a heightened immune reaction that often can lead to a leaky gut which causes other problems.

Most often than none, it's unrealistic for any lifestyle change to happen overnight. It does take practice but with practice does come change. Don't allow the bigger picture to discourage you. Every small thing you change to better your health will pay off in the end. It's the small steps that can make a big difference. Start by looking at your life and evaluating the toxins you may regularly come in contact with, understand what must take priority, and replace with these alternative options that I have listed in this article.

You have the power to make a difference in your life. You've always had the power. No one can force you to become more aware of what you put on your body and what you put in your body. What you eat is just as important as what you put on your body. Adjusting your life, reading labels and catering to your specific health needs isn't easy but it will benefit you in the long run. This is one of the smartest decisions that you can make. Not only will you start to look and feel better but think of the medical cost that you could be saving your future self.

Healthy Cells Grow From the Inside Out

Look into getting a Knowledgeable Health Practitioner:

The very first thing that you need to do is look into getting a knowledgeable holistic health practitioner!

The main reason why you should work with a knowledgeable health practitioner is its patient-centered medical healing at its best. Unfortunately, when it comes to your body there isn't a one size fits all approach to dealing with it and often times you are left still searching for the answers to your symptoms when all you want is your zest for life back. A knowledgeable health practitioner will care for you as an individual as they won't look at your body as a whole they will treat each individual body symptom, imbalance and dysfunction. They will take into consideration the whole person, including physical, mental and spiritual aspects, when treating a health condition or promoting wellness. I want you to understand that you are made up of interdependent parts and if one part is not working properly, all the other parts will be affected. A knowledgeable health practitioner certainly moves from the confusion of the "one size fits all treatment" approach that we know isn't working to the one that will cater to what your body needs. Let's not forget that each of us are a unique case and unless you get a proper thorough clinical evaluation, trying to figure what medical advise you need online is dubious at best.

In order to find your food code here are a list of things that need to be addressed in your life. When all these things are addressed and you are learning to know what your body needs and needs to avoid then you can find your personal food code. I never said it was going to be easy.

1. Address Food sensitivities

Food allergies

Many people are unaware that certain foods are actually working against their bodies. You should see a specialist and be tested to ensure you have no food allergies. Your lymphatic system can also be affected by your gut. If your gut is inflamed and not healed this is taxing on your immune system which in return is taxing on your lymphatic system. Consider adding prebiotics and probiotics to help support gut health along with eating properly and avoiding these common food allergens.

Common food allergens that can contribute to an inflamed gut are:

Nightshades

Eggs

Grains (gluten)

Dairy

If you allergic to certain foods it is will involve you're the immune system. You know that your immune system controls how your body defends itself. Your body see's inflammatory foods as invaders and will kick in your autoimmunity responses.

For example if you have a food allergy to cow's milk, your immune system will see cow's milk as an invader. In-return your immune system overreacts by producing antibodies called Immunoglobulin E (IgE). These antibodies travel to cells that release chemicals, causing an allergic reaction to start fighting for your body. Being tested for food allergies seems to be easiest way to check to see if you have any food allergies so you can start avoiding these foods and help your immune system become strong again.

2. Address nutritional deficiencies

Having nutritional deficiencies certainly adds gas to the fire. When you are deficient it can aggravate the symptoms: vitamin D, iron, omega-3 fatty acids, selenium, zinc, copper, vitamin A, the B vitamins, and iodine.

3. Address Chronic Candida

Did you know that an overload of Candida was picked up at birth or shortly thereafter? We were supposed to be getting good friendly bacteria from our mother's at birth, but "our" mother's had Candida overgrowth and unknowing passed it on to us. And over the years, our bodies has become more and more compromised. Your gut microbes could be dramatically affecting your thyroid health. There is a lot of misinformation and misunderstanding about Candida. Both from the medical profession and on the internet. It is easy to get fooled into thinking, as many sites will try to convince you, that all anyone needs to do is to take their product or buy their e-book. Of course, they will all have testimonies. What they don't tell you in those testimonies is how the Candida came back — in a month or two or in six months. However long it took for the Candida to overgrow enough to start causing symptoms again. It is important to know that dealing with Candida is not an easy fix.

4. Address Hormonal imbalances

After researching many hours on this topic, I've found that where your body stores fat is hint to what is going on with you internally with your hormones. As our hormone levels change with age, pregnancy, exercise, eating habits, or other life events, fat adjusts itself to our every changing hormonal events and places itself in different area's in our body. Our hormones have a direct impact on how much body fat we store and where it is stored on our bodies. Wouldn't it be wonderful to know what approach to take to fix those thunder thighs or that muffin top? Now even with this information it's just a stepping stone of knowledge to better equip you a healthier you. This completely changes how you and what you should be eating.

So what exactly does it mean to have fat stored in certain areas of your body and not others?

Love handles/belly: Love handles often means that you are way too stressed out and when you're stressed out it raises your cortisol levels. It could also be an indicator that you might have adrenal fatigue. Cortisol adds fat around my mid-section. You are eating too much sugar where you become insulin resistant. If your body is in constant elevated levels of insulin (a hormone that regulates the metabolism of carbohydrates in the bloodstream) it will accumulate around your mid-section. A lack of sleep also may lead to metabolic issues and help encourage those love handles. It also could mean you have elevated estrogen levels and more insulin production. So what do you need to do? Stop eating crap, those processed carbs and avoid sugar, even the fake sugars which are even more horrible for you. You should also go easy on the exercise, sometimes if you exercise more it adds more cortisol to your body so you are fighting a losing battle, try yoga, more sleep, meditation, Pilates, planks, lifting weights and walking are good ways to start. Don't forget fat gained around the waist is dangerous in terms of it increases the risk of heart disease, diabetes and other chronic diseases.

Thighs: Sometimes it's our genetic bone structure that was passed down from our parents that gives us more hips or fatter thighs than the next person and other times it can mean that we have elevated estrogen levels. This is the female sex hormone. Thigh fat is a little harder to burn off than belly fat. You can also have fluid retention in your thighs. So many think that fluid retention only takes place only in the abdomen but that isn't true It actually occurs all over your body. So what do you need to do? Start drinking your daily needed allowance of water. Your body weight and divide it by two. That's the least amount of water to drink per day and please don't drink it all in one sitting. There is a think called water toxicity and it will kill you. Space out your water consumption. Choose better skin care products in my blog 21 Successful Tips on Clean Beauty Swaps. I share with your skin care products are healthier. You want to avoid chemicals such as BPA (that can be found in plastic containers, water bottles and pretty much anything plastic unless it states BPA FREE), parabens or phthalates. Your food should be 100% organic and you most defiantly should be avoiding all soy products like the black plague. Let's not forget that getting in a good night's sleep will also help to improve your estrogen levels.

Back of Arms: This could mean that you have lower testosterone levels as well as an excess insulin. Women do have a small amount of testosterone in our adrenal glands and ovaries although this is thought as a male hormone. Start eating more avocados, as in healthy fats and fatty fish such as salmon can help improve this area. Try to avoid all red meat and all dairy products. Start trying to lift some weights. Building muscle through weight lifting can and may also increase testosterone levels.

Upper Back: This could mean you have lower levels of Thyroxine and higher levels of insulin. Thyroxine is a thyroid hormone that plays a role with your metabolism and calorie burning rate and this hormone is secreted into our bloodstream. You can help boost your thyroxine naturally by eating foods such as shellfish, seafood and cruciferous vegetables, avoiding gluten and soy, and increasing healthy fat intake.

Our metabolism does not decide to burn or store body fat based on calories. It makes these decisions based on the hormones those calories trigger. That is why the quality of calories matters so much….higher-quality calories trigger body-fat-burning hormones while low-quality calories trigger body-fat-storing hormones.

Body fat is important necessity for life. It is our source of energy and it stores some much needed nutrients, a major ingredient in brain tissue. Moreover, it provides a padding to protect internal organs and insulates the body against the cold. But yet, getting too fat (more than 30 percent body fat in females and 25 percent in males) can be dangerous and is associated with increased risk of disease and premature death, regardless of where the fat is stored in the body. As a American society, we are tipping the scales to the point that obesity is now a national health epidemic.

Here are some other factors that contribute to estrogen dominance:

    Eating clean. Let's talk about eating clean whole nutrient rich foods. Start reading label. If you must eat prepacked foods always look for foods that have a short ingredient list and things that are recognizable as actual food. Various chemicals are added like sugars, questionable oils, and sodium and so on. Always avoid soy and if soy is listed as an ingredient. Soy comes in all varieties and are highly processed, high in refined starches, heated oils and again added sugar, salt and low in nutrients and fiber. Oh let's not fail to mention that soy mimics your hormones and plays a very sneaky trick on your endocrine system.

Poultry or beef raised on hormones. Although it may cost a little bit extra try to eat free-range or grass-fed animals that are raised without hormones and antibiotics.

Chemicals found in consumer products Personal care products loaded with parabens, petroleum, and phthalates. Did you know that products we use every day may contain toxic chemicals and has been linked to women's health issues? They are hidden endocrine disruptors and are very tricky chemicals that play havoc on our bodies. "We are all routinely exposed to endocrine disruptors, and this has the potential to significantly harm the health of our youth," said Renee Sharp, EWG's director of research. "It's important to do what we can to avoid them, but at the same time we can't shop our way out of the problem. We need to have a real chemical policy reform." The longer the length of ingredients on your food label means how much more unhealthy it is for you to consume. When an item contains a host of ingredients that most likely you can't even pronounce or remember to spell you can bet your lucky dollar that the natural nutrients are long gone. These highly processed frank n foods are very difficult for the body to break down and some of the chemicals will become stored in your body. Click on this link to see what you should avoid.

You can also find many great DIY personal care recipes alternatives in my book, **AWARENESS HAS MAGIC**. Here are three recipes from my book **AWARENESS HAS MAGIC**.

Lemon Cream Body Butter

6 Tablespoons coconut oil

¼ cup cocoa butter

1 Tablespoon vitamin E oil

3 drops of Lemon essential oil or 3 drops of your favorite essential oil

Over low heat in a double boiler, put the coconut oil and cocoa butter in a bowl. When it has almost completely melted, remove from the heat and add the vitamin E oil and essential oil. Allow the mixture to cool until it solidifies. Lastly mix the body butter vigorously with a spatula, and then transfer it to a mason jar with a sealable lid. Date and label your product. If you don't care for the lemon essential oil, use whatever smells best to you. This is your journey not mine I am only here to help guide you.

Homemade Shaving Cream

1 cup shea butter

1 cup virgin coconut oil

3 Tablespoons vitamin E oil

3 Tablespoons sweet almond oil or olive oil or jojoba oil

3 Tablespoons Dr. Bonners Liquid Castile Soap

30 drops of lavender essential oil (optional)

30 drops of lemon essential oil (optional)

I like to use an electric mixer, mixing all ingredients until stiff peaks are formed (approximately 2-3 minutes). Store in a mason jar with a sealable lid.

Mosquito Repellent

15 drops of lavender

4 tbsp. of vanilla extract

1/4 cup freshly squeezed lemon juice

Place all these ingredients in a 16oz then fill with water.

Insomnia. It's amazing how the food we eat affects our health, sleep patterns and even our "gasp" sex drives. Unfortunately, when you don't get enough sleep, it can age us faster , cause depression, weight gain, make us forget things, gives us headaches and we have a greater chance of developing heart disease. If you have issues like snoring or sleep apnea and are overweight, one thing you can do is lower your body fat index. For those of us that don't have snoring or sleep apnea we ask the question," Sleep why you hate me so much!" We need to feed our bodies to get more, Tryptophan, serotonin and melatonin. (serotonin is a brain chemical that helps you sleep) and melatonin (the hormone that makes you sleepy) Trytophan is an essential amino acid, which means you have to gt it from your diet because your body cannot produce it. Your body uses tryptophan to make the neurotransmitters serotonin and melatonin. Red Onion Tea helps with insomnia

Directions

- 1 cup of water
- 1 onion, cut in quarters
- Blend, strain and drink

Epsom salt bath which is rich in magnesium

Sleepy time Goats Milk Bath

- 2 cups of powdered goat's milk
- 2 cup of Epsom salt
- 1 cup of sea salt
- 2 cup of baking soda
- 10 drops of lavender essential oil

Combine the dry ingredients and the lavender essential oil. Store in a closed container. When you are ready to take a bath add 1 cup of dry ingredients. (Kids can use up to 1/2 cup of the mixture). Bathe 3 times weekly, soaking for at least 12 minutes.

Lavender has a reputation as a mild tranquilizer. Simply dab a bit of the oil onto your temples and forehead before you hit the pillow. The aroma should help send you off to sleep.

Lastly, don't obsess over not sleeping. Studies have shown that people who worry about falling asleep have greater trouble falling asleep! It may help to remind yourself that while sleeplessness is a pain in the ass it isn't life-threatening. Let's try to be mellow-bellow. Eat foods that foods contribute to calmness and sleepiness.

5 plants to help you sleep better!

1. Aloe Vera — emits oxygen at night to help you combat insomnia and improve the overall sleep quality.

2. Lavender- Lavender is a plant that is well known to induce sleep and reduce anxiety. The smell of lavender slows down your heart rate and reduces anxiety levels.

3. Jasmine plant- The smell of jasmine has been shown to improve the quality of sleep.

4. English Ivy- it's beneficial for those who have breathing problems and asthma. Studies have shown that English ivy can reduce air molds to 94% in 12 hours.

5. Snake plant- emits oxygen into the night while you sleep, taking carbon dioxide from the air inside your home. It also filters nasty household toxins from the home.

Poor liver function due to the use of pharmaceuticals drugs. You really need to do research on your medications. Some medications have a negative effect on your lymph system and since estrogen is metabolized primarily in the liver try to not use pharmaceutical drugs unless absolutely necessary. If you must take these medications then try introducing liver-supporting supplements into your diet, such as cucumber juice, milk thistle extract, calcium d-glucarate, folic acid and taurine.https://www.lymphnet.org/membersOnly/dl/reprint/Vol_24/Vol_24-N4_Drugs_LE.pdf

Magnesium deficiencies Magnesium is necessary for metabolizing estrogen in the liver. Magnesium is a mineral that plays an important part in our health and well-being. It's one of the forgotten minerals and it's vital for many processes within the body. Magnesium helps to keep the nervous system healthy and to calm your nerves when you are stressed. In fact, did you know that magnesium is the first mineral depleted when you are stressed? So if you have any type of stress in your life magnesium is the first mineral that goes out the window. Magnesium is also an important mineral co-factor for enzymes that have biochemical reactions in the body. In other words it plays a large role in digestive system health as it helps enzymes do their job as well as to loosen the body to relax and ease to support the metabolic processes. These recipes are from my book AWARENESS HAS MAGIC.

Calming Magnesium Body Butter My homemade magnesium body butter will help replace the magnesium that our bodies need to thrive to survive. I always try to apply a little to my feet and shoulders before bed. This helps me relax and also get a fantastic night's sleep. It's pretty easy to make and the benefits are overwhelming. Magnesium deficiency is very common and it mimics other common symptoms and many other conditions like, being tired and felling run down, not sleeping well, getting headaches, gut issues, and even feeling stressed and anxious. Here is a list of things that can lower our magnesium levels:

Too much caffeine

Processed food and Sugar

Too much stress

Poor sleep habits

Calming Magnesium Body Butter

1/2 cup cocoa butter

1/2 cup of coconut oil and melt

1/4 cup magnesium oil

Add 10 drops of lavender essential oil,

Add 10 drops cedarwood essential oil

Add 10 drops frankincense essential oil

Place a heat-safe glass measuring cup/bowl inside a pot that has 1-2 inches of simmering water over medium heat. Add the cocoa butter and melt it in your double boiler until it's completely melted.

Remove the cocoa butter from heat, and add 1/2 cup extra virgin coconut oil to the melted cocoa butter and stir until completely the coconut oil has melted. Next add 1/4 cup magnesium oil to the mixture and combine. Place the mixture in the refrigerator to cool for about 30-60 minutes (until it is cooled completely). After the mixture has completely cooled and became a solid. Use a hand mixer or stand mixer to whip it. Start on low and increase speed slowly. Whip for about 3-5 minutes. Next add the 10 drops each of lavender essential oil, the 10 drops of cedar wood essential oil, and the 10 drops of frankincense essential oil. Scrape down the sides of the bowl and continue whipping for another 5 minutes or so, until the magnesium body butter is light and fluffy. The color of the magnesium body butter will change from yellow to a pale ivory and almost white color. Lastly put the magnesium body butter into mason jars and seal tightly with a lid. Make sure to label and date the top of the lid. This recipe makes enough for two 4 oz. glass jars.

Did you know that it takes 26 seconds for the chemicals to enter into your bloodstream? The real reality is we are damaging our DNA and we are changing our genetic makeup for future generations. There was a study a few years back that said the umbilical cord of an average American baby has over 200 known chemicals in it. Eighty percent of the common chemicals that are used daily in this country, we know almost nothing about. Our children are being born toxic and we have no idea if these toxins are already doing some sort of damage their brains, their immune system, their reproductive system, and any other developing organs. Are we unknowingly setting ourselves up for failure in the womb, even before birth?

Scientists and researchers are concerned that many of these chemicals may be carcinogenic or wreak havoc with our hormones, our body's regulating system.

Most products have a warning label that is typed in bold "Keep out of Reach of Children". As consumers, we believe that if our children don't ingest these products they will not be harmed by them. This can be far from the truth. Think about other common methods of exposure are through the skin and our respiratory tract. WE are along with our children are often in contact with the chemical residues housecleaning products do leave behind, by crawling, lying and sitting on the freshly cleaned floor.

Scientists at Norway's University of Bergen tracked 6,000 people, with an average age of 34 at the time of enrollment in the study, who used the cleaning products over a period of two decades, according to the research published in the American Thoracic Society's American Journal of Respiratory and Critical Care Medicine.

These chemicals can chemicals bind together.

Exposure to phthalates has been associated with lower IQ levels.

These chemicals can also be found in the shampoos, conditioners, body sprays, hair sprays, perfumes, make up, cleaning supplies, colognes, soap and nail polish that we use.

The results follow a study by French scientists in September 2017 that found nurses who used disinfectants to clean surfaces at least once a week had a 24 percent to 32 percent increased risk of developing lung disease.

Scientists and researchers are concerned that many of these chemicals may be carcinogenic or wreak havoc with our hormones, our body's regulating system.

It's not enough to be aware of all the outdoor chemicals that we are exposed to everyday but inside our homes we can have more power and control. We have to be more aware about using chemical cleaners, paints, glues, body lotions, toothpastes, underarm deodorants, hair products and pesticides. Instead start to begin to use products that don't pollute our very own bodies. We must read labels, make our own products and do our own research. I can't stress this enough. We must take a stand for our health. Stop using commercial products that are laced with unknown and harmful body damaging products.

You can reduce your exposure to them by eating organic foods, making your own cleaning chemicals and using alternative pest control methods.

You can also find many great recipes for alternative cleaning solutions in my book AWARENESS HAS MAGIC.

Here are two recipes from my book AWARENESS HAS MAGIC.

Vanilla grapefruit linen spray

2-1/2 cups filtered water

3 drops pink grapefruit essential oil

2 drops vanilla essential oil

1/4 cup vodka

The vodka helps the water dry quickly after you spray it on your linens. Theses essential oils that are used create a beautifully fresh vanilla grapefruit scent that is perfect for a summer pick me up. This spray is very versatile. It can be used on clothing, fabric furniture, or even as a quick air freshener.

If the vodka smell is slightly strong just add another drop or two of essential oil.

Always shake the bottle be before spraying on your linen.

Tub & Tile Cleaner

1/4 cup baking soda

1/4 cup lemon juice

Or 10 drops of lemon essential oil

3 Tablespoons Epsom salt

3 Tablespoons Sal Suds or Castile liquid soap

1/2 cup white vinegar

Pour the vinegar into the bottle, followed by the baking soda and Epsom salt. Shake the bottle to combine the ingredients. Add the Sal suds gently shaking the bottle to combine. Mix all ingredients in a bottle with a sealable lid.

Scrub and then rinse with water and wet clean rag.

5. Parasites and Heavy Metals

Heavy metals weaken our body's defense system against foreign invaders and make it convenient for them to set up house. American's are not being protected as we should from pollution. We don't have to go to a 3rd world country or even a foreign country be subjected to contaminated water which can led to illnesses. The pollution in our air, water, food supply, cleaning products, body products, commercial weed killers and chem trails in our environment. It's really hard not to have some sort of health issues that come from a heavy metal over load on our bodies. Just imagine commercial meat production, can goods and prepackaged foods. Heavy metals make a very acid environment which is very harmful to your gut flora where parasites and candida love to flourish. Candida and parasites actually do serve a purpose in your body they are to protect us from the potentially fatal complications of heavy metal poisoning. They feed on heavy metals and store them within biofilms- buffering us from heavy metal overload.

Do you find that you are developing new allergies as you become older; are you always tired, do you have poor digestion, gas, heartburn; sugar cravings, are you irritable, frequent headaches; poor memory, "fogged in" feeling, dizziness, recurring depression, vaginal infections, menstrual difficulties, urinary tract infections, infertility, hay fever, postnasal drip, habitual coughing, catch colds easily, sore throat, athlete's foot, skin rash, psoriasis, cold extremities, arthritis-like symptoms, do you feel miserable in general? If answered yes to most of these symptoms then should be tested for candidiasis.

According to the publication in 1995 "Parasitic Diseases" it states the following rate of infection per species.

Nematodes (Round Worms)	1 billion individuals
Cestodes (Tape Worms)	300 million individuals
Tremadodes (Flukes)	300 million individuals
Protozoa (Amoebas)	1 billion individuals
Arthropods (Insects parasites)	500 million individuals

How can I start to detox from Parasites and Heavy Metals?

Each per-son is different and I encour-age you to seek out a qual-i-fied nutri-tion-ist or other qualified healthcare practitioner in order to assess exactly which nutri-ents, herbs, homeopathic and nat-ural reme-dies and/or in which com-bi-na-tion that will help you achieve your goal. No one treatment is the same since we all have different diary needs, illness's and lift styles. Getting the root cause of your issues are the main objective. I strongly recommend you get with your health care provider and allow them to schedule you for further tested if needed. This is how and where you will figure your own personal food code.

6. Heal your Gut

Your gut is your portal to health. It houses 80 percent of your immune system, and without your gut being healthy it is practically impossible to have a healthy immune system. A leaky gut have been linked to hormonal imbalances, autoimmune diseases such as rheumatoid arthritis and hashimotos thyroiditis, diabetes, chronic fatigue, fibromyalgia, anxiety, depression, eczema and rosacea, and that is just to name a few. So you can understand why a properly working digestive system (your gut) is vital to your health. Contrary to what we use to believe. We now know that having a leaky gut is one of the main reasons, and probably the beginning stage, for developing an autoimmune disease. Having a leaky gut means that the tight junctions that usually hold the walls of your intestines together have become loose, allowing undigested food particles, microbes, toxins, and more to leave your gut and enter your bloodstream. This will cause your body to become full of inflammation, which in return will start to trigger an autoimmune condition and if you already have an autoimmune condition it will certainly make it worse. Luckily for you. Your gut is made up of wonderful cells that can turn over very quickly, so you can start to heal your gut in as little as thirty days, by following these 4 R guidelines: Remove, Restore, Replace and Repair

Remove the damage — Remove these inflammatory foods, household & body chemicals, drink filtered water(to avoid fluoride and chloride) , stop using aluminum brand deodorant, start using fluoride free brand tooth pastes, start to reduce your stress that damage your gut, do a detox to heal any gut infections from yeast, parasites, or bacteria.

Restore the Strong — replenish the enzymes and digestive acids that are necessary for proper digestion

Replace with friendly Bacteria — Make sure you are taking plenty a good strong probiotic that is full of these much needed "good bacteria" to start supporting your immune system. Here is a great product that I use. You can do your own research and I am sure there are other brands out there that are wonderful too. Garden Of Life Dr. Formulated Probiotics Once Daily Women's, 30 Count

Repair the digestive Tract — Give you gut a fighting chance by supplying the nutrients and amino acids needed to build a healthy gut lining. (Gelatin can improve your ability to produce adequate gastric acid secretions that are needed for proper digestion and nutrient absorption. Glycine from gelatin is important for restoring a healthy mucosal lining in the stomach and facilitating with the balance of digestive enzymes (Here is a brand that I use   Garden of Life RAW Enzymes Women, 90 Capsules) and stomach acid. The best way to consume gelatin make them into broth or soup. You can do this by simply brewing some bone broth at home using this Bone Broth Recipe.

Hypothyroidism Foodies: Tips on how to be successful in the kitchen

When you are starting to eat to cater to your hypothyroidism or Hashimoto's disorder, every meal seems to be a challenge. Once you start to eliminate all grains, processed foods, caffeine, soda's, fake food and any food allergens you seem to be left with what can I eat? Each week I decide what I am going to eat. I like to plan ahead. I like easy & fast. Since my kids have all grown up and it's normally me here alone in the evenings, cooking for one is rather boring and I am honestly, burnt out from cooking all these years.

We are creating a perfect storm within our bodies. The less nutrients we consume, more toxins we add, create this world win of health issues. It's sad that our western diet is made up of red meats, vegetable oils, white flour and sugar. Who would have thought that something so simple as eating has become so complicated? Food does matter. It talks to your DNA. Food can change your DNA!

The foods you eat have a major impact on autoimmune disease — It affects your gut health and along with increasing or decreasing the inflammation in your body. Unfortunately, our western world diet are full of foods that have a bad impact on both your gut and your inflammation.

We've been molded and brain washed with the American standard diet. You see, there are so many healthy options possible and available at your fingertips that if you know what you can eat all you have to do is google recipes for that food item and create your own dish. Have google and imagination, will travel, right? Please don't feel this is complicated. It's not.

Do a little research and you will find that our western diet that is made up of processed, fake foods, chemicals, sugar and corn oils are all highly flaming the fan of your inflammation. Begin to start reading labels. You will soon discover that health foods such as low-fat and gluten-free packaged foods, which are often loaded with sugar, additives, and preservatives. Avoid Grains, dairy, legumes, eggs, corn, and soy which these foods are not the cornerstones to a healthy diet anymore they can contribute to a leaky gut and inflammation.

Tips on how to be successful in the kitchen!

1. Never skip breakfast!

   Keeping your blood sugar stable throughout the day is important. You don't want your blood sugar to drop nor get to high. Eating breakfast does jump-start your digestion and fire up your metabolism, as well as helping the body regulate blood sugar levels. Also, when you skip breakfast it makes your adrenal glands respond by secreting a hormone called cortisol. Cortisol then tells the liver to produce more glucose, bringing blood sugar levels back to normal. What happens when you have too much cortisol? It collects around you midsection. With hypothyroidism you already have higher levels of cortisol in your body than someone without hypothyroidism. Cortisol is that hormone that is involved in the "flight or fight" response. Before you go grab that donut or high carb breakfast remember the word, metabolic syndrome. There is a strong connection between thyroid dysfunction and metabolic syndrome. Metabolic syndrome is caused by chronic hyperglycemia (high blood sugar). When you gobble down too many carbs, the pancreas secretes insulin to move excess glucose from the blood into the cells where glucose is used to produce energy. But over time, the cells lose the ability to respond to insulin. After so long of your insulin knocking at your front door of the cells. The cells stop hearing them. The pancreas responds by pumping out even more insulin (knocking louder) in an effort to get glucose into the cells, and this eventually causes insulin resistance. So with all this being said how should you handle breakfast with hypothyroidism?

Never skip it

Wait 1 hour after you have taken your thyroid medication and wait 4 hours after your thyroid medication to take any supplements. Also, if you take other medications check with your pharmacists to make sure it's okay to take it along with your thyroid medications.

Drink lemon water with your thyroid medication. It cleanses the digestive system and gets your metabolism firing on all cylinders.

Pick a low GI and healthy protein with a healthy fat for breakfast. I love eggs and I am not allergic to them but many are. I eat 2 boiled eggs, sauerkraut along with a tablespoon of coconut oil (healthy fat) and a splash of organic apple cider vinegar in my decaf green tea. This is your breakfast. Be creative. Low GI fruits and veggies will help you not have sugar spikes! Eating a low-glycemic foods will help you control your calories, eat high-fiber, high-nutrient foods, and help you manage your weight more successfully. Sample breakfast for you could be gluten free old-fashioned oats, a tablespoon of flax-seed oil or coconut oil, cinnamon healthy fat and blueberries. Another breakfast option is 2 slices of nitrate free uncured turkey bacon or nitrate free, uncured bacon along with avocado and blueberries.

Option #3: Greek Yogurt/nondairy yogurt or Cottage Cheese topped with berries and almonds.

Option #4: Can of Tuna, organic Apple and 1tbs of olive oil

Option #5: organic Chicken breast, organic Salad Greens, Apple and Half an Avocado

Option #6: cage free Omelets, 2 whole eggs and Berries cooked in a good fat

Option #7: Garden of life fit shake mix with 1 cup unsweetened almond milk, 1 tablespoon of flax-seed oil and serving of blueberries

Another smoothie recipe is
Half of Avocado

1 handful organic romaine lettuce

1 handful of organic celery

1 handful of organic cucumber

1/2 cup of blueberries

8 ounces of water, blend and drink......

Since we are talking breakfast try to hit the re-bounder for at-least 5 minutes too. A rebounder is great for getting your lymph fluid flowing and keeping your thyroid healthy. The lymphatic system and thyroid play a big part in your metabolic rate, so getting them moving is a great option.

Meditation

Start your day out with meditation and a grateful heart. There are many people who weren't able to wake up and live another day. I can't even begin to express the importance of the power of meditation has over the body. It's been proven to lower your levels of cortisol which is also known as the stress hormone. I like to start my day off listening to mediation music to clear my head while I have my legs up against the wall using this yoga pose.

Legs up the wall pose will not only help with your thyroid functions but it also relieves back pain, helps with insomnia, improves posture, helps with anxiety, naturally adjusts your spine, improves your digestion and it starts a lymphatic circulation. Your lymphatic system doesn't have a pump and relies on our movements and gravity to circulate lymph fluid where the toxins in this fluid can be eliminated from your body. If we sit all day the lymph fluid becomes stagnant and start to collect toxins. By simply reversing the flow of gravity in your legs, you begin to circulate the lymphatic fluid and encourage the body to start the elimination of toxins. Dry brushing also will simulate the lymphatic system and improve skin tone.

2. Meal prepping

On Sunday I always meal prep because it helps improve my time management throughout the week, helps keep me stay on track, saves me money, helps me regulate my portion control , helps me stay mentally in the game and has been the #1 one strategy that has helped me eat healthy meals and snacks throughout the week . Since this food task has already been complete I don't worry about what I am going to eat. I can open up the fridge and grab what I need. Meals stored in the fridge will usually last three days. I never chance it further than that others do.

3. Leftovers are wonderful

Sometimes you just don't feel like cooking the next day. There is nothing wrong with eating dinner for breakfast the following day. Sometimes you just get so busy that you barely have time to think. Let alone have time to meal prep for the week. You're short on time so how about cooking meals that work double-time and I personally think taste even better after sitting a day in the fridge.

4. Try Batch cooking.

Batch cooking to me runs on the same lines as meal prepping but your freezing these meals to grab later and cook. This also can help you stay on track with hypothyroidism diet by being prepared. A simple way to always have food ready is to batch cook. When you batch cook you spend a little longer in the kitchen by preparing a big load of food that you can warm-up the following days.

5. Slow cooking

 I love coming home to mouthwatering smells of a homemade ready to eat slow-cooked meals! All you have to do is grab a plate and dig in.

Hashimoto's crock-pot recipes: Added Bonus: How I put my Hashimoto's into remission

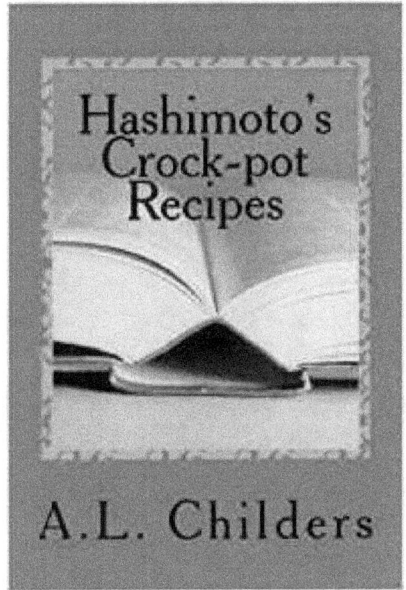

There's nothing like the aroma of a home-cooked dinner welcoming you at the door. No time to be in the kitchen? The wonderful thing about a crock pot is you have little prep time. You won't have to stand over a hot stove cooking your food and it's perfect for those hectic days. We all want that convenience! Do you need foods that promote thyroid health? You can start today healing your body from the inside out. Over 101 wholesome and nourishing Hashimoto's fighting recipes that will cater to your mind, body and soul. This helpful book will start to guide you in the right direction along with a step by step plan that is clear and doable.

It's not about being skinny, it's about energy, vitality & feeling good when you look in the mirror.

Kicking Hypothyroidism's booty, The Slow Cooker way: 101 Slow Cooker recipes!

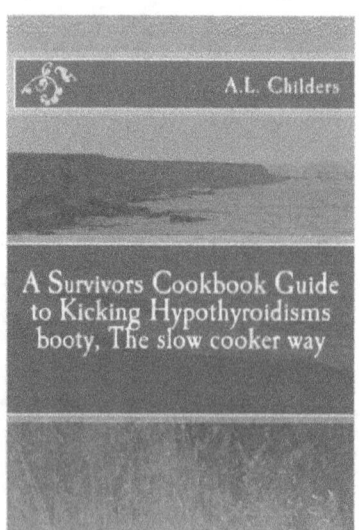

I wanted to create a user-friendly handbook to help anyone affected by this disorder. I've seen many doctors over the years and none offered me ideas on diet change. I've included recipes, ideas on solutions for a healthier home, what you should be eating and shouldn't, how to shed those extra pounds, regain your self-confidence and vitality back into your life. I want you to feel strong, sexy, and beautiful. This is my heartfelt guide to you. Together, once again, you can start to gain that wonderful life that you deserve. I am a student in this thing called life. I want to be remembered as a pioneer who thought, imagined, and inspired. What we feel at times is the impossible or unthinkable. Life is a wonderful journey.

6. Address Food sensitivities

Food allergies

If you allergic to certain foods it is will involve the immune system. You know that your immune system controls how your body defends itself. Your body see's inflammatory foods as invaders and will kick in your autoimmunity responses. For example if you have a food allergy to cow's milk, your immune system will see cow's milk as an invader. In-return your immune system overreacts by producing antibodies called Immunoglobulin E (IgE). These antibodies travel to cells that release chemicals, causing an allergic reaction to start fighting for your body. Being tested for food allergies seems to be easiest way to check to see if you have any food allergies so you can start avoiding these foods and help your immune system become strong again.

7. Fix your gut

Probiotics can help to begin repairing the lining in your gut. This also aids in helping to balance your hormones. if someone has leaky gut syndrome it allows undigested food particles to leak through your gut into your bloodstream and in return creates disease-causing inflammation that will have a impact on your body — especially your thyroid glands where they are very susceptible to inflammation. Did you know that your gut is the largest component of your immune system? It introduces friendly bacteria into your digestive system that helps to keep illness's at bay and they are rich in live bacteria that help us absorb nutrients along with maintain proper microbiome gut balance. Research has proven that gut health could affect inflammation, allergies and autoimmune disorders in the body as a whole. Around 1,000 different species of bugs live in your gut. Your gut has been linked to contributing to weight loss and for overall improvement of numerous symptoms, including depression, anxiety, brain fog, skin problems, hormonal issues, immune weaknesses, digestive problems, and fatigue.

Gut-Healing Vegetable Broth

- 12 cups filtered water
- 1 tbsp. coconut oil
- 1 red onion, peeled and cut in half
- 1 garlic bulb smashed
- 1 chili pepper roughly chopped
- 1 thumb-sized piece of ginger roughly chopped
- 2 cups of watercress
- 3-4 cup mixed chopped vegetables and peelings I used carrot peelings, red cabbage, fresh mushrooms, leeks and celery
- 1/2 cup dried shiitake mushrooms
- 1/4 of a cup dried wakame seaweed
- 1 tbsp. peppercorns
- 2 tbsp. ground turmeric
- 1 tbsp. organic apple cider vinegar
- A bunch of fresh parsley

Simply add everything to a large pot. Bring to a boil then simmer, with the lid on, for about an hour.

Once everything has been cooked down, strain the liquid into a large bowl.

Natural Probiotics

There are different types of probiotics. Some are pills, powders, or capsules that contain billions of live bacteria and will help to replenish your microbiome. Fermented foods are more of a nature type of probiotic. They carry live bacteria plus many other crucial nutrients. Many cultures all around the world has its own recipes for fermented foods.

Garden Of Life Dr. Formulated Probiotics Once Daily Women's, 30 Count

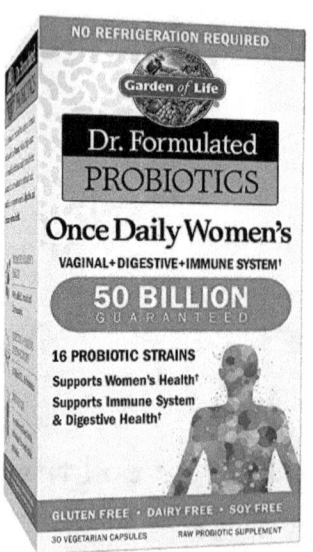

8. Detox your lifestyle

We are creating a toxic shit storm within our very own bodies. I'm not speaking from a place of Prejudice or judgement because what you do with your life is entirely your call. The real reality is we are damaging our DNA and we are changing our genetic makeup for future generations. Did you know that most of these products we use every day contain toxic chemicals and has been linked to women's health issues? They are hidden endocrine disruptors and are very tricky chemicals that play havoc on our bodies. "We are all routinely exposed to endocrine disruptors, and this has the potential to significantly harming our health. Start making your own cleaning products. My book Awareness has Magic is full of DIY nontoxic cleaning recipes along with body recipes.

Recipes

21 days of Hypothyroidism Shakes

Breakfast is the most important meal of the day. Breakfast" literally means the meal that "breaks the fast". You've been sleeping all night fasting. Your body needs to be rebooted. You've got to "jump-start" that metabolism. Eating a healthy breakfast has been medically proven to have many health benefits, including weight control , reducing the risk of obesity , it certainly will boost your fiber intake to help you reach your daily goal of 20 to 35 grams (for adults). Eating breakfast has been shown to improve performance, have heart health advantages, helps you avoid fluctuating glucose levels, which can lead to diabetes later in life, helps you consume less calories throughout the day, so you're not binge eating of starvation at lunch time. It will give you that mental edge by enhancing your memory, your clarity, and the speed in which you are processing information, your reasoning skills, your creativity and how you absorb information. Scientists at the University of Milan in Italy reviewed 15 studies and found some evidence that those benefits. One theory suggested that if you eat a healthy breakfast it can reduce hunger throughout the day, and help you make better food choices at other meals. You should eat no later than 2 hours of waking up. Also, if you skip breakfast your hunger hormones are boosted and it can also throw your body into survival mode. Which in return starts breaking down protein in your muscles and your muscles will slowly start to break down. I hope you understand and see the importance of why eating a healthy breakfast is so important.

Be creative with your smoothies. If they are too thick, add more liquid, if they are too thin for your liking add less liquid. Play with the ingredients. This is your 21 day reboot. Make a smoothie that you know you're going to drink. Every single smoothie has celery in it. The reason why celery is in every smoothie is it has super health benefits that range from reducing inflammation, regulates the body's alkaline balance, aids digestion, reduces "bad" cholesterol, reduces bloating, helps to prevent ulcers, lowers blood pressure, amps up your sex life, cancer fighter, excellent source of antioxidants and beneficial enzymes, in addition to vitamins and minerals such as vitamin K, vitamin C, potassium, folate and vitamin B6.

I also suggest that you go with an all-natural vegan, gluten free, dairy free, lactose free, no fillers, no synthetic nutrients, no artificial flavors or sweeteners, no preservatives , no pea protein and soy free protein mix. This is why I use Raw Meal, Garden of life brand products. No they are not endorsing me to say this. I picked this brand after a long research. I am sure there are other brands just as good as this brand but I prefer this brand.

Become mindful and read labels. You want to stay clear of hidden poisons that can be in your protein powders. Here are 3 to be on the lookout for to avoid.

Soy Protein Isolate

Soy protein has been a main ingredient in many protein powders for a while. Soy has been found to be toxic to the digestive system and creates the following concerns:

Disrupts thyroid and endocrine function

Interferes with leptin sensitivity which can cause metabolic syndrome

Throws off estrogen and testosterone balance

Blocks the body's ability to access key minerals like iron, zinc, calcium, and magnesium

It is also estimated that soy is over 95% genetically modified, and one of the most pesticide ridden crops on the market.

This makes any non-organic soy protein (especially isolate) found in protein powders, indigestible and toxic to the human physiology.

Whey Protein Isolate

Whey protein can be a quality protein. Not many on the market are good to digest. If whey came from conventionally raised cows that have been fed non-organic grains and genetically modified foods, and been injected with antibiotics and hormones, which makes it not a good quality source of protein. You also need to keep in mind that this form of whey in an isolate format is not properly absorbed by the body.

If you do choose a whey protein, it is important to see where the whey has come from. Make sure it is from grass fed cows. Which are nutritionally superior compared to grain fed, and they contain an impressive amino acid and immune-supportive nutrient profile.

Rice Protein

Same as the source of the whey protein, the kicker is where it comes from. Even though rice protein can be an acceptable source of protein but many that are not.

Thanks to a report unveiled earlier in 2014 by Mike Adams, we have been able to discover that there are many rice protein powders on the market that have been heavily contaminated with tungsten, cadmium, and lead. The reason for this high level of contamination is due to sourcing rice from China, where air pollution can trump the "organic" label placed on many products, including rice.

Super Charge Green Smoothie

½ organic cucumber, chopped

2 celery stalks

¼ cup parsley

½ lemon, peeled

½ avocado, peeled and pitted

2 cups of organic romaine lettuce

1 scoop of raw meal- garden of Life

1 cup of coconut water

1 cup of ice

Add all ingredients to blender and blend until smooth. Enjoy!

Blueberry Chocolate Delight

½ cup of frozen blueberries

1 cup of romaine lettuce

2 celery stalks

½ teaspoon of Ceylon Cinnamon

1 scoop of raw meal –garden of life- chocolate flavor

2 tablespoons of almond butter

1 cup of unsweetened nut milk

Add all ingredients to blender and blend until smooth. Enjoy!

Happy Colon Smoothie

1 cup pumpkin puree

2 stalks of celery

1 tablespoon raw honey

½ of a peeled grapefruit

1 cup unsweetened almond milk

2 tablespoon flaxseed meal

½ inch fresh raw ginger

½ teaspoon cinnamon, nutmeg & turmeric

This a delicious, easy drink to make. Add all ingredients into the blender and voila!

Green Boosting Smoothie

1 cup mixed baby greens

½ avocado, peeled and pitted

2 organic celery stalk

½ cucumber

2 springs of parsley

1 cup coconut milk

1 scoop of raw meal-garden of life

Add all ingredients to blender and blend until smooth. Enjoy!

Seaweed-Me Green Smoothie

1/2 cup Organic Kelp, chopped

1 Organic Apple, sliced

2 celery stalks

1/2 Organic Avocado

1 cup Coconut Water

1 scoop of raw meal-garden of life

½ cup of ice

Add all ingredients to blender and blend until smooth. Enjoy!

****Keep in mind that many hypothyroidism cases are actually caused by Hashimoto's thyroiditis. It was found in some research that increasing iodine intake could actually cause your thyroid issues to worsen if you have Hashimoto's. Instead, reducing iodine intake may be the solution. If you have Hashimoto's, please check with your health care provider before adding any iodine to your diet. Organic Kelp is loaded with natural Iodine.

Simple Pina Colada Smoothie

1 cup of Organic Pineapple

1 cup of Coconut Milk

2 celery stalks

1 tablespoon of raw, unprocessed, unfiltered coconut oil

1 tablespoon of ground flaxseed

1 tablespoon of spirulina

½ cup of ice

Add all ingredients to blender and blend until smooth. Enjoy!

Alamo Splash Smoothie

1 orange, peeled & deseeded

1 cup of fresh pineapple

2 celery stalks

Juice from 1 lime

½ avocado, peeled & pitted

1 cup of coconut water

1 tablespoon of ground flax seed

1 tablespoon of spirulina

½ cup of ice

Add all ingredients to blender and blend until smooth. Enjoy!

Bahama Mama Smoothie

1 whole lemon, peeled and deseeded

1 cup of pineapple, chunked

2 celery stalks

1 cup of green tea (or my favorite Matcha green tea)

1 tablespoon of ground flax seed

1 tablespoon of spirulina

½ cup of ice

Add all ingredients to blender and blend until smooth. Enjoy!

Coconut Shake-me Smoothie

1 cup of unsweetened coconut milk

½ inch fresh ginger, peeled

2 celery stalks

1 teaspoon of Ceylon cinnamon

2 tablespoons of almond butter

½ cup of shredded unsweetened coconut flakes

1 scoop of vanilla flavored raw meal-garden of life

½ cup of ice

Add all ingredients to blender and blend until smooth. Enjoy!

Flaming Flamingo Smoothie

1 cup 100% organic cranberry juice

2 celery stalks

1 cup pineapple, diced

1 whole lemon, peeled and seeded

1 tablespoon of ground flax seed

1 tablespoon of spirulina

½ cup of ice

Add all ingredients to blender and blend until smooth. Enjoy!

Sexy and Sassy Smoothie

½ cup of frozen blueberries

½ teaspoon of Ceylon cinnamon

2 celery stalks

1 tablespoon of almond butter

1 cup of tonic water

1 tablespoon of ground flax seed

1 tablespoon of spirulina

½ cup of ice

Add all ingredients to blender and blend until smooth. Enjoy!

Citrus Apple Sensation

½ frozen peeled avocado

1 cup apple, cored and diced

2 celery stalks

1 cup fresh romaine lettuce

1 handful of fresh parsley

½ lemon, juice squeezed into the blender

1 cup filtered water

Add all ingredients to blender and blend until smooth. Enjoy!

Blueberry Booster Smoothie

1 cup blueberries

1 medium banana, peeled

1 cucumber, peeled and cut up

1 cup of filtered water

1 tbs chia seeds

This a delicious, easy drink to make. Add all ingredients into the blender and voila!

Before Sunrise Glee

1¼ cups almond milk

2 celery stalks

½ cup of soaked oats

1 fresh apple, cored and diced

¼ tsp cinnamon

1/2 cup cherries

1 scoop of raw meal- garden of life

Add all ingredients to blender and blend until smooth. Enjoy!

Polka Dot Berry Dance

1½ cup almond milk

2 celery stalks

1 tbsp. chia seed powder

1 handful fresh romaine lettuce

1/3 cup frozen blueberries

Add all ingredients to blender and blend until smooth. Enjoy!

Green Royal Colada

1 large cucumber

2 celery stalks

½ cup of kefir water

½ cup fresh parsley

½ cup pineapple

½ cup ice

1 tablespoon of coconut oil

1 tablespoon of ground flax seed

1 tablespoon of spirulina

Add all ingredients to blender and blend until smooth. Enjoy!

Green Watermelon Monster

1 cup watermelon, diced

2 celery stalks

½ cucumber

2 tablespoons of ground flax seed

1 tablespoon of Dulse flakes

1 teaspoon of spirulina

Add all ingredients to blender and blend until smooth. Enjoy!

Super Green Women Smoothie

1 cup unsweetened almond milk

2 celery stalks

1 cup of romaine lettuce

1 tablespoon of almond butter

1 tablespoon of coconut oil

1 teaspoon of spirulina

1 cup of frozen mixed berries

1 tablespoon of ground flaxseed

½ cup ice

Add all ingredients to blender and blend until smooth. Enjoy!

Blueberry Shake Me Smoothie

1 cup frozen blueberries

2 celery stalks

1 cup romaine lettuce

1 cup of coconut milk

½ avocado, peeled and pitted

1 tablespoon of chia seeds

½ teaspoon of cinnamon

1 scoop of raw meal-garden of life

Add all ingredients to blender and blend until smooth. Enjoy!

Chocolate cherry Butter Ginger Shake

1 cup unsweetened chocolate almond milk

2 celery stalks

½ inch fresh ginger, peeled

½ cup frozen cherries

1 tablespoon coconut oil

1 teaspoon of Ceylon cinnamon

1 tablespoon of almond butter

1 scoop of chocolate raw meal- garden of life

Add all ingredients to blender and blend until smooth. Enjoy!

Green Berry Bomb Smoothie

1 cup of romaine

2 celery stalks

½ cup frozen berry mix

1 cup light coconut milk

2 tablespoon of gluten free old fashion oats

1 tablespoon honey

Add all ingredients to blender and blend until smooth. Enjoy!

I wanted to give you a surprise. Not everyone likes smoothies. I've added a few extra healthy hypothyroidism friendly breakfasts.

Basic overnight oats

1/3 cup GF steel cut or rolled oats (steel cut for a crunch or rolled oats for a smoother oatmeal)

1/3 - 1/2 cup almond milk or coconut milk [depending on how thick you like it]

1/3 cup plain So Delicious Greek style yogurt

1/2 banana, mashed

1/2 tbsp. chia seeds (Omega 3 fatty acids)

½ Teaspoon ground cinnamon

Directions

Stir everything together in a bowl. Put in a mason jar with lid. Refrigerate for at least 6 hours, preferably overnight.

Almond butter and Banana Overnight Oats

1 large ripe banana, mashed (about ½ cup)

¼ cup creamy almond butter

1 cup GF steel cut or rolled oats (steel cut for a crunch or rolled oats for a smoother oatmeal)

1 cup unsweetened almond milk

1 tablespoon chia seeds (optional) (Omega 3 fatty acids)

½ teaspoon vanilla extract

½ teaspoon ground cinnamon

1 teaspoon raw honey

In a medium bowl, mash your banana with a fork.

Add the remaining ingredients to the bowl and mix until well combined.

Pour the mixture into two 8 oz. mason jars with lids, seal tightly and Refrigerate for at least 6 hours, preferably overnight. When ready to eat, give the oats a good shake and dig in!

Almond Butter Chocolate Overnight Oats

1/2 cup GF steel cut or rolled oats (steel cut for a crunch or rolled oats for a smoother oatmeal)

1 tsp chia seeds

1 tsp flax meal

2 tsp cacao powder

1 T almond butter

1 chopped medjool date or 2 tsp grade B maple syrup

1/2 cup almond milk

Directions:

Pour the mixture into a 8 oz mason jars with lids, seal tightly and Refrigerate for at least 6 hours, preferably overnight.

When ready to eat, give the oats a good shake and dig in!

No-bake oatmeal bites

1 cup dry quick oats

2/3 cup coconut flakes

1/2 cup almond butter

1/2 cup dark chocolate chips

1/3 cup raw honey

1 tsp vanilla

Directions: Mix all ingredients, form into 1 inch balls. Place balls in refrigerator and this is a quick and easy fast just grab n go healthy breakfast option.

Chickpea, tomato and Zucchini Frittata

Eggs are among one of the healthiest foods on the planet. Eggs are particularly rich in the two antioxidants Lutein and Zeaxanthine. Eggs are loaded with high-quality proteins, vitamins, minerals, good fats and various trace nutrients, 6 grams of protein with all 9 essential amino acids. Rich in iron, phosphorous, selenium and vitamins A, B12, B2 and B5. Make sure to purchase omega 3 rich eggs, free roaming & organic not factory raised. Not all eggs are created equal. Stay away from your standard supermarket eggs. The chickens are usually raised in an overfilled hen house or a cage and never see the light of day. They are usually fed a grain-based feed that are supplemented with vitamins and minerals, antibiotics and hormones. So Like the commercial states it really is the incredible, edible egg!

Ingredients:

2 Tbsp. coconut oil or olive oil

1 onion, thinly sliced

1 zucchini, thinly sliced

½ cup of cherry tomatoes cut in half

1 (15-oz.) can chickpeas, drained

1 garlic clove, crushed

½ tsp. chili flakes

½ tsp. ground cumin

3 Tbsp. chopped flat leaf parsley

6 organic cage free eggs

Directions:

Heat oil in a cast iron skillet. Add onion and sauté over medium heat for 6-8 minutes or until golden brown.

Add zucchini and tomatoes, increase the heat and sauté for 4 minutes or until softened. Stir in chickpeas, garlic, chili flakes, cumin and parsley and stir-fry for 2 minutes or until hot. Beat eggs with 2 tablespoons water and stir into vegetables. Place in oven and cook on 350 for about 20 minutes until its set.

Smoked Salmon Frittata

Eggs, salmon, and tomatoes. This recipe is loaded with all the nutrients that you need. The eggs have disease-fighting nutrients like lutein. Your salmon is loaded with omega 3's, a good source of protein, B vitamins, vitamin D, magnesium and selenium. The tomatoes are also a powerhouse of nutrients from vitamin C, biotin, molybdenum, and vitamin K , copper, potassium, manganese, dietary fiber, vitamin A (in the form of beta-carotene), vitamin B6, folate, niacin, vitamin E, and phosphorus. Sounds like a perfect meal for breakfast or brunch.

Ingredients:

3 eggs

2 ounces smoked salmon

1 roma tomato, diced and seeded

¼ cup chopped onion

½ tablespoon chopped parsley leaves

1 tablespoon goat's milk

2 tablespoons olive oil

Celtic Salt and pepper to taste

Method:

Preheat the oven to 350 °F.

Break the eggs in a bowl, add goat's milk and seasoning, and whisk them.

Heat the oil in a cast iron skillet. Sauté the onions till golden brown, add the diced tomato and add seasoning. Add the salmon and sauté for 2 additional minutes. Pour the egg mixture in the pan and stir gently. Place in the preheated oven and cook for 20-25 minutes.

Homemade Turkey Sausage Patties

Turkey is rich in protein, low in fat and is a source of iron, zinc, potassium, phosphorus, vitamin B6 and niacin. It also contains the amino acid tryptophan, selenium and is lower on the GI index scale.

1 lb of ground turkey

1 teaspoon of dried sage

½ teaspoon of fennel seeds

Dash of cayenne, black pepper and ground all spice

Mix all ingredients in a bowl. Shape into small 3 inch patties and allow to refrigerate for 2 hours to help form. In a cast iron skillet on medium heat, cook the patties until completely cooked through on both sides. This would be great with some freshly scrambled eggs.

Honey-lime Fruit Salad

This easy-to-make breakfast is full of vitamins and antioxidants

Ingredients:

2 cups chopped seasonal fruits (I use red grapes, kiwis, mandarins, and bananas)

1 teaspoon lime juice

1 tablespoon organic honey

Directions:

Combine all the ingredients in a mixing bowl.

Breakfast Quinoa with Blueberries

Quinoa is naturally gluten-free and contains iron, B-vitamins, magnesium, phosphorus, potassium, calcium, vitamin E and fiber. Quinoa is a health food superstar. This ancient grain is one of only a few plant foods that are considered a complete protein and has all essential amino acids. Quinoa is a slowly digested carbohydrate, naturally high in dietary fiber so this makes it a great low-GI option and an awesome choice for diabetics! Can you believe it!?

Ingredients

1/2 cup of dry quinoa, rinsed

1 cup of unsweetened vanilla almond milk

1/2 teaspoon of vanilla extract

2 tablespoons of almond butter

½ teaspoon Cinnamon

½ cup of organic Blueberries

Directions:

Add quinoa, almond milk and vanilla extract to a saucepan and bring to a boil. Lower heat and simmer with cover on until liquid is absorbed. Fluff quinoa with a fork and let sit uncovered for about a minute.   Mix in almond butter, cinnamon and the blueberries.

Apricot Squares

2 c gluten free old fashion oats

¼ c ground flaxseed

¾ tsp ground cinnamon

¼ tsp ground cloves

¼ tsp Celtic or Himalayan salt

½ c almond butter

¼ c raw honey

1 tsp vanilla extract

½ c finely chopped apricots

PREHEAT your oven to 350°F. Coat your 8" x 8" pan with spray.

1st mix the dry ingredients in a bowl. Next, mix the wet ingredients in a separate bowl. Add to the dry ingredients and your wet ingredients and mix to combine. Mix in the apricots until well combined. PRESS the mixture firmly into your prepared pan. BAKE for 25 minutes, or until the edges are browned. Let it cool completely before cutting into eight bars.

Slow Cooker Apple Cranberry Steel Cut Overnight Oats

2 cups gluten free steel cut oats

1 Tbsp. raw honey

1 1/2 cups fresh cranberries

3/4 cup unsweetened organic applesauce

2 apples, peeled, cored and sliced

1/4 cup coconut sugar

1/2 tsp Celtic sea salt

1/4 tsp pure vanilla extract

3 cups unsweetened vanilla almond milk

3 cups water

Spray your crock pot with non-stick spray Put all the ingredients into your slow cooker and cook overnight on low for 8 hours). Once cooked, stir oats to combine and serve. Ladle into your bowl and serve.

Slow Cooker Toasted Granola

½ cup honey

½ cup applesauce

¼ cup organic coconut oil

¼ cup of almond butter

1 teaspoon of ground Ceylon cinnamon

5 cups of gluten free rolled oats

½ cup raw pumpkin seeds

2 teaspoons of ground flaxseed

½ cup organic golden raisins

¼ cup chopped pitted dates

Spray slow cooker with a nonstick spray. In a small bowl whisk together honey, applesauce, oil, almond butter, and cinnamon. In the slow cooker add the combine oats, pumpkin seeds, and flax seeds. Stir in honey mixture. Cook on high-heat setting about 2 1/2 hours or until toasted, stirring every 30 minutes. Allow the lid to vent. After its finished cooking. Spread the oat mixture on a pan to cool. Add raisins and dates; toss gently to combine. Store in an airtight container at room temperature for up to 5 days or freeze for up to 2 months. Ladle into a bowl and serve.

Slow Cooker Hearty Breakfast Quinoa

1 cup Quinoa

2 cups apple juice

1/4 teaspoon Ceylon cinnamon

1/8 teaspoon nutmeg

½ apple, diced

2 tablespoons real maple syrup (grade B)

1/4 cup dried cranberries

Spray your slow cooker with non-stick spray. In a mesh strainer, rinse out the quinoa for about 3 minutes. Combine the quinoa, apple juice, cinnamon, and nutmeg, diced apple, maple syrup and dried cranberries into the slow cooker. Mix well. Cook on low for 6-7 hours or until liquid has been absorbed.

Fermented Apple Sauce

6-8 red organic apples

2 tablespoons of water kefir

1 teaspoon of cinnamon

½ teaspoon of Himalayan sea salt

Core and slice apples. Blend in a food processor, add your kefir, cinnamon and salt.

Pour apple sauce into clean mason jars and seal with the lids. Leave about an inch of space from the apple sauce to the lid of the jars. (Might explode if not) Store in your food dehydrator for 3 days on the lowest warm tempura available. 100 F. Next place it in your fridge and make sure you eat it within two months.

Recipes

21 days of Hypothyroidism Salad-in-a-Jar Lunches

Some of the recipes call for Greek yogurt. If you prefer not to eat cow's milk dairy yogurt. I have a recipe for homemade nondairy coconut yogurt in the back of the book or if you store carries nondairy coconut milk yogurt that is always an option too.

Healthy Hypothyroidism salads are made with leafy greens and non-starchy vegetables that are excellent for fast lunches and busy days. Theses dressings has superb taste and is made with much needed healthy fat: olive oil is high in heart-healthy monounsaturated fatty acids and MCT oil will help you kick-start fat loss. Just store it in the fridge up to 1 week and just drizzle over your favorite crunchy lettuce, tomatoes and other seasonal veggies.

Lemon Tart

Ingredients (makes 6 servings, about ¾ cup)

   ¼ cup mayonnaise

   1 tbsp. Dijon mustard

   ¼ cup extra virgin olive oil

   2 tbsp. MCT oil

   2 cloves garlic

   2 tbsp. fresh lemon juice

   2 tbsp. freshly chopped herbs of choice (parsley, oregano, basil, chives, etc.)

   Salt and pepper to taste (I like pink Himalayan salt)

Suggestions for additional seasoning and substitutions:

½ garlic powder instead of crushed garlic (organic crushed garlic is healthier)

¼ tsp chili powder or 1-2 tsp freshly chopped chili pepper

1 tbsp. Sriracha

Other healthy oils instead of olive oil, organic unrefined coconut oil, avocado, macadamia or walnut oils

Peel and chop the garlic. Place the mayo, lemon juice, garlic, mustard, finely chopped herbs (I used parsley), olive oil and MCT in a blender, blend until blended. Season with salt and pepper to taste. Next place in a jar with a covered sealed lid. Store in the fridge for up to a week. Shake well before drizzling over salads.

Garlic Salad Dressing

Ingredients

    4-6 Cloves garlic

    1/2 Cup Organic Apple Cider Vinegar

    1 Cup extra virgin olive oil

    1/3 Cup Water

    1 Tbsp. Dijon mustard

    1/4 Tsp pink Himalayan salt

    1 Pinch Black Pepper To taste

    (Optional) Fresh herbs (I used parsley)

Add all ingredients in a blender and store in a sealed mason jar.

Pomegranate Vinaigrette

Ingredients

    2 Tbs. pure pomegranate juice

    1 Tbs. raw organic apple cider vinegar

    10 cherry tomatoes

    1 tsp maple syrup (or alternative natural sweetener, like raw honey)

Instructions

    Blend together until smooth. Pairs nicely with a house salad loaded with vegetables and topped with pomegranate seeds, or coconut bacon.

Ginger Grapefruit Turmeric Glaze

Ingredients

    Juice of 1 grapefruit

    Juice of 1 inch fresh ginger root

    Juice of 2 inches fresh turmeric root, or $\frac{1}{2}$ tsp ground turmeric spice

    3 fresh dates, pitted

Instructions

    Blend together until smooth. Pairs nicely with a mixed lettuce salad topped with garlic and herb quinoa.

Creamy Avocado Lemon Dressing

Ingredients

1 ripe avocado

Juice from ½ a lemon

½ tsp pink Himalayan salt

¼ tsp cayenne pepper

½ clove of garlic, pressed

1 tsp unsweetened almond milk

Instructions

Mix together with a fork until smooth. Pairs nicely with a "Caesar" style salad for a healthy alternative to a cream based dressing.

Add cucumber and coconut bacon to top.

Chickpea Veggie Salad-in-a-Jar

This fills one 32 oz. Mason jar. Make sure to wash & dry your veggies before using.

1 oz. goat cheese

½ cup cooked, cold quinoa

1 bell pepper, chopped

1 cucumber, chopped

4 oz. grape or cherry tomatoes

5 oz. chickpeas, rinsed & dried

Dressing:

3 tsp olive oil

1 tsp white vinegar

Splash of lemon juice

Sprinkle of black pepper

Whisk dressing in a small bowl, then transfer to the bottom of the jar. Layer chickpeas on dressing. Add tomatoes, add cucumber, add bell pepper, add quinoa and top with goat cheese. Secure lid on tightly until ready to eat. Shake the salad just before eating.

Layered Quinoa Salad-in-a-Jar

This fills one 32 oz. Mason jar. Make sure to wash & dry your veggies before using.

3 Tbsp. avocado cilantro-Lime Vinaigrette

½ cup black beans, rinsed & dried

¼ cup cherry tomatoes

½ of a green pepper, chopped

½ cup cooked, cold quinoa

¼ cup organic romaine lettuce

Place the dressing in the bottom of the jar. Next add the black beans, add the tomatoes, add the peppers, add the quinoa and then add the chopped romaine. Try not to pack it in too tight, or you won't have room to shake the dressings when you are ready to eat. Seal the lid on & store in the fridge. When ready (with the lid on) shake the jar to mix everything.

Avocado Cilantro Lime Vinaigrette

½ cup extra-virgin olive oil

1 cup cilantro

¼ tsp of minced garlic

The juice of 1 orange

The juice of 3 limes

1 avocado

Salt & pepper to taste

Combine all ingredients into a blender or food processor .Puree until smooth.

Mediterranean Quinoa with Seasonal Vegetables Salad-in-a-jar

This fills one 32 oz. Mason jar. You could divide this up into smaller jars. Make sure to wash & dry your veggies before using.

1 cup quinoa, rinsed well

2 cups vegetable broth

1 zucchini, diced

1 cup of corn

½ cup cherry tomatoes, diced

¼ cup red onion, diced

Vinaigrette:

2 teaspoons whole grain mustard

3 tablespoons freshly squeezed lemon juice

1 tablespoon Bragg's organic apple cider vinegar

2 garlics clove, finely minced

1/4 teaspoon crushed red pepper flakes

Freshly ground black pepper to taste

1/2 cup extra-virgin olive oil

Roast zucchini and onions, uncovered, for 20 minutes. Stir vegetables and add tomatoes and corn. Continuing roasting until tomatoes collapse, about 10 minutes. Remove vegetables and set aside

Vinaigrette

In a medium bowl whisk together mustard, lemon juice, Braggs vinegar, garlic, red pepper flakes, salt and pepper. Gradually whisk in olive oil.

Place 3 tablespoons of the dressing in the bottom of the mason jar.

Next place the roasted cooled veggies on top of the dressing and add the quinoa. Try not to pack it in too tight, or you won't have room to shake the dressings when you are ready to eat. Seal the lid on & store in the fridge. When ready (with the lid on) shake the jar to mix everything.

Roast chicken Salad-in-a-jar

This fills one 32 oz. Mason jar. Make sure to wash & dry your veggies before using.

3 Tbsp. balsamic Vinaigrette

½ cup button mushrooms, sliced

¼ cup cherry tomatoes

½ of a red onion, minced

½ cup cooked, cold roasted chicken, diced

¼ cup organic romaine lettuce

Place the dressing in the bottom of the jar. Next add the mushrooms, add the tomatoes, add the onions, add the roast chicken and then add the chopped romaine. To make it easier on me, I buy a whole, hot roasted chicken from the deli at my local grocery store. Try not to pack it in too tight, or you won't have room to shake the dressings when you are ready to eat. Seal the lid on & store in the fridge. When ready (with the lid on) shake the jar to mix everything.

Balsamic Vinaigrette

3 tablespoons balsamic vinegar

1 tablespoon Dijon mustard

1 garlic clove, minced

1/2 cup olive oil

Salt and freshly ground pepper

In a small bowl, combine the vinegar, mustard, and garlic. Add the oil in a slow steady stream, whisking constantly. Season with salt and pepper to taste.

Layered Taco Salad-in-a-jar

This fills one 32 oz. Mason jar. Make sure to wash & dry your veggies before using.

¼ cup cucumber, diced

1 roma tomato, diced

½ cup black beans, rinsed and drained

¼ cup corn

¼ red bell pepper, diced

¼ cup avocado, diced

1 cup of romaine lettuce, chopped

2 tablespoon of goat cheese

Cilantro-lime dressing

1 tablespoon apple cider vinegar

Juice from 1 lime

½ cup fresh cilantro

¼ cup nonfat Greek yogurt (I have a recipe for nondairy yogurt in the back)

1 teaspoon raw honey

Blend the salad dressing until smooth and pour it in the bottom of your mason jar. Next layer you salad from heaviest to lightest. Add your cucumbers, then your tomatoes, next your black beans and your corn. On top of that place your red bell pepper, next your avocado. Lastly place your lettuce and then the cheese on top of that. Try not to pack it in too tight, or you won't have room to shake the dressings when you are ready to eat. Seal the lid on & store in the fridge. When ready (with the lid on) shake the jar to mix everything.

Grilled Chicken, Beet, Apple Salad-in -a-jar

This fills one 32 oz. Mason jar. Make sure to wash & dry your veggies before using.

1 beets, scrubbed, peeled and diced into small bite size pieces

1 teaspoon olive oil

Salt and pepper to taste

¼ cup roasted chicken breast, diced

1/2 apple, washed and diced

2 cups organic romaine lettuce

1 ounce goat cheese

¼ cup raw pumpkin seeds

Strawberry Vinaigrette

1/4 cup fresh strawberries

1/2 tablespoon olive oil

1/2 tablespoon balsamic vinegar

Pinch of salt

Pinch of ground black pepper

1/4 teaspoon raw honey

Blend the salad dressing until smooth and pour it in the bottom of your mason jar. Next layer you salad from heaviest to lightest. Add your beets, then your chicken and your diced apples. Lastly place your lettuce, next the goat cheese, then your raw pumpkin seeds. Try not to pack it in too tight, or you won't have room to shake the dressings when you are ready to eat. Seal the lid on & store in the fridge. When ready (with the lid on) shake the jar to mix everything.

Smoked Salmon Salad-a-Jar

This fills one 32 oz. Mason jar. Make sure to wash & dry your veggies before using.

¼ cup smoked salmon, diced

¼ cup cucumbers, diced

2 carrots shredded

¼ cup red onion, diced

2 cups organic romaine lettuce

Lemony vinaigrette

3 tablespoons olive oil

1 tablespoon white balsamic vinegar

1/2 Meyer lemon, zested and juiced

In a small bowl, whisk together olive oil, vinegar, lemon juice, and of lemon juice with the zest. Pour in the bottom of your mason jar.

Next add the cucumbers, carrots, red onion, salmon and lettuce. Try not to pack it in too tight, or you won't have room to shake the dressings when you are ready to eat. Seal the lid on & store in the fridge. When ready (with the lid on) shake the jar to mix everything.

Mediterranean Salad-in-a-jar

This fills one 32 oz. Mason jar. Make sure to wash & dry your veggies before using.

4 quarters of artichokes, canned

2 each grape tomatoes, sliced in half

1/4 cup English cucumbers, quartered and thinly sliced

1/4 cup canned Cannellini beans

1 Tbsp. goat's milk cheese crumbles

2 Tbsp. Kalamata olives, sliced

1.5 cups mixed greens

1 Tbsp. unsalted roasted sun flower seeds

Sweet red wine vinaigrette

1/2 cup red wine vinegar

6 Tbsp. water

2 Tbsp. olive oil

2 tsp. honey

1 tsp. Dijon mustard

1/2 tsp. salt

1/4 tsp. black pepper

1 tsp. oregano

1/2 tsp. basil

In a small bowl, whisk together olive oil, vinegar, honey, Dijon mustard, salt, pepper, oregano and basil. Pour in the bottom of your mason jar.

Next add the artichokes, tomatoes, cucumbers, cannellini beans, olives, lettuce, sunflower seeds and lastly the cheese. Try not to pack it in too tight, or you won't have room to shake the dressings when you are ready to eat. Seal the lid on & store in the fridge. When ready (with the lid on) shake the jar to mix everything.

Smoked Turkey Salad-in-a-Jar

This fills one 32 oz. Mason jar. Make sure to wash & dry your veggies before using.

3 tablespoons of raspberry balsamic vinaigrette

¼ cup smoked turkey, diced

¼ cup cucumbers, diced

¼ cup cherry tomatoes, diced

2 boiled eggs, diced

5 tbsp. Walnuts, raw

2 cups organic romaine lettuce

Raspberry Vinaigrette Dressing

1 cup of fresh raspberries

¼ cup olive oil

2/3 cup balsamic vinegar

1 tablespoon of honey

Blend everything until smooth.

Pour 3 tablespoons of the vinaigrette in the bottom of your mason jar. Next add your cucumbers, cherry tomatoes, turkey, romaine lettuce, boiled eggs and walnuts. Try not to pack it in too tight, or you won't have room to shake the dressings when you are ready to eat. Seal the lid on & store in the fridge. When ready (with the lid on) shake the jar to mix everything

Tuna salad-in-a-Jar

This fills one 32 oz. Mason jar. Make sure to wash & dry your veggies before using.

1 (2.6 oz.) Pouch - albacore Tuna

¼ cup diced canned artichoke hearts

¼ cup sweet baby peas

½ cup diced red and yellow pepper

¼ cup cucumber, sliced and diced

¼ cup goat cheese

2 cups chopped lettuce leaves

Pour your dressing in the bottom of jar. Layer ingredients in jar, starting with wettest ingredients at the bottom and ending with lettuce on top. Try not to pack it in too tight, or you won't have room to shake the dressings when you are ready to eat. Seal the lid on & store in the fridge. When ready (with the lid on) shake the jar to mix everything

Dressing

2 tbsp. olive oil

3 medium garlic cloves, pressed

1 tbsp. Dijon mustard

1 tsp honey

4 tbsp. lemon juice

1/4 cup ground flax seeds

Dash Italian herbs

Whisk all ingredients together

Zucchini Noodle Salad with Quinoa Salad-in-a- jar

1/3 cup cooked quinoa

2 tsp minced cilantro

1.5 tsp coconut flakes

3 asparagus stalks, chopped into 1" pieces

1/4 cup green peas

1 medium zucchini, Blade C

2-3 scallion stalks, diced

1/4 cup goat cheese

Avocado lime dressing

1/2 avocado

2 tbsp. coconut milk

Juice of 1/2 lime

Bring a small saucepan filled halfway with water to a boil. Then, add in the asparagus. 1 minute later, add in the peas. Cook for 3-4 minutes or until vegetables are cooked and pour out into a colander. Allow to cool.

Blend the dressing until smooth and place in bottom of the jar.

Next add the zucchini noodles, your quinoa mixture and the scallions. Place on top the cooled asparagus & peas. Lastly the feta. Try not to pack it in too tight, or you won't have room to shake the dressings when you are ready to eat. Seal the lid on & store in the fridge. When ready (with the lid on) shake the jar to mix everything

Marinated White Bean Salad-in-a-jar

This will make 4 pint-sized mason jars.

    1 can (19 ounces) cannellini beans, rinsed and drained

¼ red onion, diced

½ cup grape tomatoes, halved

2 cups of romaine lettuce

For the Marinated White Bean Salad:

    1 small garlic clove, minced

    1 tablespoon white wine vinegar

    1 teaspoon chopped fresh thyme

    1/2 teaspoon grated lemon zest

    1/4 teaspoon dry mustard powder

    1/4 teaspoon kosher salt

    1/8 teaspoon ground black pepper

    1/8 teaspoon red pepper flakes

    2 tablespoons extra virgin olive oil

In a bowl, whisk together garlic, vinegar, thyme, lemon zest, mustard powder, salt, black pepper and red pepper flakes. While whisking, slowly drizzle in oil until all oil is incorporated. Add beans and toss to combine.

Divide Marinated White Bean Salad equally among 4 pint-sized mason jars. Layer onion, tomatoes and romaine. Try not to pack it in too tight, or you won't have room to shake the dressings when you are ready to eat. Seal the lid on & store in the fridge. When ready (with the lid on) shake the jar to mix everything

Asparagus Tossed Salad-in-a-jar

2 medium carrots, diced into small bitesize pieces

½ cup fresh asparagus, cut into 1-inch pieces

2 celery stalks, diced

2 cups torn Bibb lettuce

ORANGE GINGER VINAIGRETTE:

1/4 cup orange juice

4-1/2 teaspoons olive oil

1 tablespoon Braggs apple cider vinegar

1 tablespoon honey

1/2 teaspoon Dijon mustard

1/4 teaspoon ground ginger

1/4 teaspoon grated orange peel

1/8 teaspoon salt

In a large saucepan, bring 4 cups of water to a boil for 1 minute. Add asparagus; cover and boil 3 minutes longer. Drain and immediately place vegetables in ice water; drain and pat dry.

Place 3 tablespoons of dressing in the bottom of the jar. Next add the asparagus, then the carrots, celery and next the lettuce. Try not to pack it in too tight, or you won't have room to shake the dressings when you are ready to eat. Seal the lid on & store in the fridge. When ready (with the lid on) shake the jar to mix everything.

Mediterranean Turkey Meatballs salad-in-a-jar

¼ cup Cucumbers, diced

¼ cup Tomatoes, diced

¼ onion Red onions, diced

4 Turkey meatballs, cooked and diced

¼ cup Artichokes, drained and chopped

¼ cup goat cheese

1 cup Romaine lettuce, diced

Zesty Italian Vinaigrette

3 Tablespoons Braggs apple cider vinegar

1 small squirt of Dijon mustard

¼ cup olive oil

½ tsp onion powder

1-2 cloves finely minced garlic

½ tsp each of thyme, basil and oregano

Salt and pepper to taste

Whisk until blended.

Pour the dressing in the bottom of the Mason jar. Next start laying it from heaviest to lightest ending with the lettuce and feta cheese on top. Try not to pack it in too tight, or you won't have room to shake the dressings when you are ready to eat. Seal the lid on & store in the fridge. When ready (with the lid on) shake the jar to mix everything.

Easy Turkey meatball recipe: 1 lb. ground turkey, 1 egg, 1/2 cup seasoned gluten free bread crumbs, 1 tsp chopped onions, 1/4 tsp garlic powder, 1/8 tsp black pepper, 1 tbsp. tomato paste. Preheat oven to 400 degrees. Combine all the ingredients and mix thoroughly. Form meatballs from 1 tbsp. of mixture mold into the shape of a ball. Bake 15 to 20 minutes on a lightly oiled 10 x 15 x 1 inch pan, or until the meatballs are no longer pink in the center. You can freeze what you don't use for later use.

Zucchini Noodle Caprese Salad-in-a-jar

¼ cup of organic chickpeas, rinsed and drained

½ organic zucchini, spiralized

½ organic tomato, diced

¼ cup red onion, diced

½ cup diced fresh mozzarella

Balsamic Vinaigrette

1 tablespoon Dijon mustard

2 tablespoons balsamic vinegar

¼ cup extra virgin olive oil

Rinse and drain the chickpeas. Place your peas in a bowl and mix ½ teaspoon each garlic and onion powder to season. Place your zucchini in a spiralizer. Squeeze the excess water out of the zucchini with a cheesecloth, kitchen towel or your hands.

In a bowl whisk your vinaigrette dressing and pour in the bottom of your mason jar. Next add the chickpeas, the zucchini, tomatoes, red onion and top with the fresh mozzarella. Try not to pack it in too tight, or you won't have room to shake the dressings when you are ready to eat. Seal the lid on & store in the fridge. When ready (with the lid on) shake the jar to mix everything.

Burrito Bowl salad-in-a-jar

This will make 4 small jars or 2 large jars.

1 cup Bob's Red Mill Tricolor Quinoa, cooked

2 grilled boneless, skinless chicken breasts, cut into bite-sized pieces

1 (14-ounce) can black beans, rinsed and drained

1 (14-ounce can) corn, drained or 1 1/2 cups fresh corn or frozen and thawed corn

2 vine tomatoes, diced

1 small red onion, diced

1 jalapeno, seeded and diced

1/2 cup chopped fresh cilantro, plus additional for serving

1 large avocado, diced

Dressing

1/4 cup extra virgin olive oil

1/4 cup freshly squeezed lime juice, plus additional for serving

1 teaspoons ground chili powder

1 teaspoon ground cumin

1/2 teaspoon kosher salt

1/4 teaspoon cayenne pepper

1/4 teaspoon black pepper

Cook the quinoa according to the package instructions. Allow to cool once done. Whisk together the dressing ingredients in a small bowl. Evenly Place the dressing in the bottom of the jars. Next start to layer your jar. Place the chicken, quinoa, black beans, corn, tomatoes, red onion, and cilantro.

Try not to pack it in too tight, or you won't have room to shake the dressings when you are ready to eat. Seal the lid on & store in the fridge. When ready (with the lid on) shake the jar to mix everything.

Cajun Shrimp salad-in-a-jar

¼ cup sautéed bell peppers, diced

¼ cup sautéed onions, diced

¼ cup Cajun shrimp, cooked

¼ cup freshly smashed guacamole

½ cup Boston Bibb lettuce

Sautee your bell peppers and onions in extra virgin olive oil. Set aside. Next sauté your shrimp in dash of paprika, garlic granules, chili powder, cayenne, and Himalayan sea salt. Cook until completely pink. You want to buy shrimp that is already deveined and the tails are cut off.

Fresh-Fantastic-Super-Quick and Easy Guacamole Recipe

1 medium avocados, 1/2 firm tomato, finely diced, ¼ cup of a red onion, diced; ¼ cup of freshly chopped cilantro;1 tbsp. fresh lime juice;

Open the avocados and scoop out the flesh. An easy way is to cut it length-wise around the pit and then using a chef's knife strike the pit and then twist the knife so you can easily remove the pit and scoop out the flesh.

Mash the flesh with a fork, it can still have hard parts, stir the other ingredients.

Start layering your jar. Peppers, onions, shrimp, fresh guacamole, and lastly the lettuce. Try not to pack it in too tight, or you won't have room to shake the dressings when you are ready to eat. Seal the lid on & store in the fridge. When ready (with the lid on) shake the jar to mix everything.

Zucchini Pasta Salad-in-a-jar

1 ½ cup spiraled zucchini

½ cup sliced celery

½ cup carrot, diced

½ cup chopped red bell pepper

½ cup cherry tomatoes, diced

¼ cup feta cheese

2 tablespoons Kalamata olives

Avocado Dressing

½ ripe avocado, peeled and seed thrown away

Juice of 1 lemon

2 tablespoons extra virgin olive oil

2 tablespoons Greek yogurt, plain (I have a recipe for coconut yogurt in the back)

½ teaspoon Himalayan sea salt

¼ teaspoon pepper

In a high powdered blender mix dressing ingredients until smooth. Place in the bottom of the Mason jar. Next Spiral or shred or thinly slice zucchini. Place in the jar on top of the dressing. Add celery, the carrots, the peppers, the feta cheese, the tomatoes and the olives. Try not to pack it in too tight, or you won't have room to shake the dressings when you are ready to eat. Seal the lid on & store in the fridge. When ready (with the lid on) shake the jar to mix everything.

Chopped Cobb Salad-in-a-jar

¼ cherry tomatoes, halved

½ cucumber, sliced

¼ red onion, chopped

2 hard-boiled eggs, chopped or sliced

½ avocados, chopped

2 slices cooked crispy nitrate free turkey, crumbled

2 slices, thinly sliced turkey, cut into pieces

2 slices, thinly sliced ham, cut into pieces

1 cups chopped romaine lettuce

Ranch dressing

5 tablespoons of buttermilk (I have a recipe for nondairy butter milk in back)

3 tablespoons plain Greek yogurt (I have a recipe for coconut yogurt in the back)

1/4 teaspoon onion powder

1/4 teaspoon dried dill

1/2 teaspoon dried parsley

1/2 teaspoon dried chives

1/2 teaspoon salt

Pepper to taste

Blend dressing until smooth. Pour the dressing in the bottom of the jar. Next add tomatoes, cucumbers, onion, egg, avocado, turkey bacon, turkey, ham, and ending with romaine. Try not to pack it in too tight, or you won't have room to shake the dressings when you are ready to eat. Seal the lid on & store in the fridge. When ready (with the lid on) shake the jar to mix everything.

Romaine Salad-in-a-jar

1 cups garbanzo beans, rinsed and drained

½ cup diced tomatoes

½ diced red onion

1 cup romaine lettuce, diced

4 white mushrooms, diced

2 hard-boiled eggs, peeled and diced

Quick Salad Dressing

2 tbsp. extra virgin olive oil

4 tbsp. Braggs Apple Cider Vinegar

A pinch of salt and pepper

Blend dressing until smooth. Pour the dressing in the bottom of the jar. Next start layering form heaviest to lights ending with lettuce and boiled egg on top. Try not to pack it in too tight, or you won't have room to shake the dressings when you are ready to eat. Seal the lid on & store in the fridge. When ready (with the lid on) shake the jar to mix everything.

Southwest Salad-in-a-jar

1 C. Romaine

¼ C. black beans

¼ C. corn (fresh, frozen or canned)

1 small tomato, diced

¼ cooked chicken, diced (or cooked ground turkey)

2 green onions chopped

¼ cup shredded cheese

½ small avocado chopped

Black Olives

Dressing

¼ cup Greek yogurt (I have a recipe for coconut yogurt in the back)

¼ cup Salsa

1 tablespoon of low sodium taco seasoning

Blend the dressing until smooth and pour it in the bottom of the jar. Next Add from heaviest to lightest ending up with the romaine on top. Try not to pack it in too tight, or you won't have room to shake the dressings when you are ready to eat. Seal the lid on & store in the fridge. When ready (with the lid on) shake the jar to mix everything.

Recipes

21 days of Hypothyroidism Dinners

Along with your dinner, don't forget to drink your bone broth.

Slow Cooker Simple Bone Broth

Ingredients

3-4 lbs. of bones

1 gallon water

2 tablespoons apple cider vinegar

2 small onions, peeled and quartered

4 small carrots, cut into 1-inch pieces

4 stalks celery, cut into 1-inch pieces

1/2 bunch flat-leaf parsley

1 bunch fresh thyme

1 head garlic, halved crosswise

1 tsp. black peppercorns

Instructions

Add everything to the crockpot.

Cook on low setting in crockpot for 10 hours.

Cool the broth, strain in a mesh strainer and pour broth into container.

Store in refrigerator.

Scoop out the congealed fat on top of the broth.

Gut-Healing Vegetable Broth

12 cups filtered water

1 tbsp. coconut oil

1 red onion, peeled and cut in half

1 garlic bulb smashed

1 chili pepper roughly chopped

1 thumb-sized piece of ginger roughly chopped

2 cups of watercress

3-4 cup mixed chopped vegetables and peelings I used carrot peelings, red cabbage, fresh mushrooms, leeks and celery

1/2 cup dried shiitake mushrooms

1/4 of a cup dried wakame seaweed

1 tbsp peppercorns

2 tbsp ground turmeric

1 tbsp organic apple cider vinegar

A bunch of fresh parsley

Simply add everything to a large pot. Bring to a boil then simmer, with the lid on, for about an hour.

Once everything has been cooked down, strain the liquid into a large bowl.

Keep in mind that many hypothyroidism cases are actually caused by Hashimoto's thyroiditis. It was found in some research that increasing iodine intake could actually cause your thyroid issues to worsen if you have Hashimoto's. Instead, reducing iodine intake may be the solution. If you have Hashimoto's, please check with your health care provider before adding any iodine to your diet. Organic Kelp is loaded with natural Iodine

Spaghetti Squash & Turkey Meatballs

1 3-pound spaghetti squash

2 tablespoons water

2 tablespoons extra-virgin olive oil, divided

1/2 cup chopped fresh parsley, divided

1 1/4 teaspoons Italian seasoning, divided

1/2 teaspoon onion powder

1/2 teaspoon salt, divided

1/2 teaspoon freshly ground pepper

1 pound 93%-lean ground turkey

4 large cloves garlic, minced

1 28-ounce can no-salt-added crushed tomatoes

1/4-1/2 teaspoon crushed red pepper

Halve squash lengthwise and scoop out the seeds. Place face down in a microwave-safe dish; add ¼ cup water. Microwave, uncovered, on High until the flesh can be easily scraped with a fork, 10 to 15 minutes.

Heat 1 tablespoon oil in a large skillet over medium-high heat. Scrape the squash flesh into the skillet and cook, stirring occasionally, until the moisture is evaporated and the squash is beginning to brown, 5 to 10 minutes. Stir in 1/4 cup parsley. Remove from heat, cover and let stand.

Meanwhile, combine the remaining 1/4 cup parsley, 1/2 teaspoon Italian seasoning, onion powder, 1/4 teaspoon salt and pepper in a medium bowl. Add turkey; gently mix to combine (do not overmix). Using about 2 tablespoons each, form into 12 meatballs.

Heat the remaining 1 tablespoon oil in a large nonstick skillet over medium-high heat. Add the meatballs, reduce heat to medium and cook, turning occasionally, until browned all over, 4 to 6 minutes. Push the meatballs to the side of the pan, add garlic and cook, stirring, for 1 minute. Add tomatoes, crushed red pepper to taste, the remaining 3/4 teaspoon Italian seasoning and 1/4 teaspoon salt; stir to coat the meatballs. Bring to a simmer, cover and cook, stirring occasionally, until the meatballs are cooked through, 10 to 12 minutes more.

Serve the sauce and meatballs over the squash.

Garlic Shrimp with Cilantro Spaghetti Squash

1 2 1/2- to 3-pound spaghetti squash, halved lengthwise and seeded

2 tablespoons extra-virgin olive oil

1 tablespoon minced garlic

1 teaspoon ground coriander

1 teaspoon ground cumin

1/2 teaspoon salt, divided

1/4 teaspoon cayenne pepper

1/3 cup dry white wine

1 pound peeled and deveined raw shrimp (16-20 per pound), tails left on if desired

1 tablespoon lemon juice

1/4 cup chopped fresh cilantro

2 tablespoons non-dairy butter, melted

1/4 teaspoon ground pepper

Lemon wedges for serving

Halve squash lengthwise and scoop out the seeds. Place face down in a microwave-safe dish; add ¼ cup water. Microwave, uncovered, on High until the flesh can be easily scraped with a fork, 10 to 15 minutes. Next heat oil in a large skillet over medium-high heat. Add garlic, coriander, cumin, 1/4 teaspoon salt and cayenne; cook, stirring, for 30 seconds. Add wine and bring to a simmer. Add shrimp and cook, stirring, until the shrimp are pink and just cooked through, 3 to 4 minutes. Remove from heat and stir in lemon juice.

Use a fork to scrape the squash from the shells into a medium bowl. Add cilantro, butter, pepper and the remaining 1/4 teaspoon salt; stir to combine. Serve the shrimp over the spaghetti squash with a lemon wedge on the side.

Oven-Fried Salmon Cakes over a bed of Quinoa Pilaf

1 (14.75 ounce) can wild-caught pink or red salmon

1 cup cooked (or canned) sweet potato, mashed

2 large eggs, beaten

1/2 cup almond flour

1/2 cup fresh parsley leaves, minced (about 2 tablespoons)

2 scallions, white and green, very thinly sliced

1 tablespoon Old Bay Seasoning

1 teaspoon salt

1 teaspoon hot sauce

1/2 teaspoon paprika

1/4 teaspoon ground black pepper

Zest from 1 lemon

2 tablespoons non-dairy butter, melted

Preheat the oven to 425F and cover a large baking sheet with parchment paper. Drain the liquid from the salmon and using your fingers, crumble the fish into a large mixing bowl, removing the bones and flaking the fish. Add the sweet potato, eggs, almond flour, parsley, scallions, Old Bay Seasoning, salt, hot pepper sauce, paprika, black pepper, and lemon zest. Mix well and refrigerate for 10 minutes.

Brush the parchment paper with some of the melted non-dairy butter, then use a 1/3 measuring cup to scoop the cakes and drop them onto the parchment. The patties should be about 2 1/2 inches wide and about 1 inch thick. Brush the tops of the cakes with the nondairy butter, then bake for 20 minutes. Carefully flip each patty with a spatula and return to the oven. Bake an additional 10 minutes until golden brown and crisp. Serve with a squeeze of lemon juice and your sauce of choice.

Quinoa Pilaf

1/2 cup diced onions

1 cup white mushrooms, chopped

1 stalk celery, diced

2 cloves garlic, minced

2 tablespoons Extra-Virgin Olive Oil

1 cup Quinoa, pre-rinse

2 cups vegetable stock, low sodium

1/4 teaspoon crushed red pepper flakes

1/2 teaspoon black pepper

Salt to taste

In a large cast iron skillet, add oil, turn to medium-low heat, add white mushrooms and saute for about 3 minutes. Add onion, garlic and celery to mushrooms and continue cooking until onion and celery are tender, about 4 minutes.

Add Quinoa, red pepper flakes, black pepper and salt to taste, stir to combine. Add vegetable stock, stir and cook for 15 minutes or until liquid is absorbed.

Once quinoa is done. Lay a few scoops on a plate. Place your salmon patties on top of the quinoa pilaf and drizzle with Sriracha-Lime Mayonnaise

Sriracha-Lime Mayonnaise

6 Tablespoons mayonnaise (recipe in back for homemade mayo)

2 teaspoons Sriracha sauce

1 teaspoon grated lime zest

Stir together all ingredients and drizzle over salmon patties

Garlic Zucchini Noodles w/ meat balls

2 zucchinis, cleaned

1 tablespoon EVOO

¼ teaspoon garlic powder

¼ teaspoon garlic salt

1 pound lean ground chicken or turkey

4 large cloves garlic, minced

1 28-ounce can no-salt-added crushed tomatoes

1/4-1/2 teaspoon crushed red pepper

Pepper to taste

Spiralize your zucchini.

Meanwhile, combine the remaining 1/4 cup parsley, 1/2 teaspoon Italian seasoning, onion powder, 1/4 teaspoon salt and pepper in a medium bowl. Add ground chicken. ;

Gently mix to combine (do not overmix). Using about 2 tablespoons each, form into 12 meatballs.

Heat the remaining 1 tablespoon oil in a large nonstick skillet over medium-high heat. Add the meatballs, reduce heat to medium and cook, turning occasionally, until browned all over, 4 to 6 minutes. Push the meatballs to the side of the pan, add garlic and cook, stirring, for 1 minute. Add tomatoes, crushed red pepper to taste, the remaining 3/4 teaspoon Italian seasoning and 1/4 teaspoon salt; stir to coat the meatballs. Bring to a simmer, cover and cook, stirring occasionally, until the meatballs are cooked through, 10 to 12 minutes more.

In another skillet on the stove over medium heat.

Once pan is hot, add EVOO and zoodles. Let sauté for about a minute, then add in the seasonings. Cook additional 2-3 minutes. Zoodles should be soft, but still have a slight stiffness. Next incorporate the zoodles and the meatball/sauce mixture and gentle mix.

Cajun grilled chicken with lime black-eyed bean salad & guacamole

For the chicken breast

1 tsp coconut oil

½ tsp dried oregano

½ tsp dried thyme

1 tsp smoked or regular paprika

¼ tsp cayenne pepper

1 garlic clove, finely chopped

4 skinless, boneless chicken breast

Mix together the oil, herbs, spices and garlic in a large resealable bag. Put the chicken breasts in the bag and mix thoroughly to cover. Bash the chicken with the side of a plate to thin it out some, then set aside to marinate for at least 15 mins.

Oil your grill then turn the heat on. Place the chicken breasts on it and grill for 10 mins, checking occasionally. Once golden brown, turn and grill for a further 5-7 mins. Check the middle of the breasts after 5 mins and, if no longer pink, and the juice looks clear, remove from the heat.

The black-eyed bean salad

1 can of black-eyed peas, drained

2 tomato, diced

1 cup of frozen sweetcorn, thawed

2 spring onion, diced

2 roma tomatoes, diced

Zest and juice 1 lime

$\frac{1}{2}$ teaspoon of ground coriander

In a large bowl, mix all the ingredients for the bean salad. Mix well and set aside.

For the guacamole

1 avocado, peeled and pitted

$\frac{1}{4}$ red chili, deseeded and finely chopped

$\frac{1}{2}$ tbsp. olive oil

Juice 1 lime

For the guacamole, scoop the flesh from the avocado and put it in a medium bowl, mash it with a fork until it the preference texture you like. Add the rest of the ingredients and mix well.

Place 1 warm chicken breast on each plate, with some bean salad and a scoop of the fresh guacamole on the side.

Maple Glazed Grilled Salmon

2 tablespoons Grade B pure Maple Syrup

3 tablespoons dark Balsamic Vinegar

2 raw Salmon fillets, with the skin on

Sea Salt and Black Pepper to taste

1 tablespoon Olive Oil

Combine balsamic vinegar and maple syrup in a resealable bag. Seal the salmon fillets in the bag and marinate for at least 10 minutes (or longer, if you have time) while you prepare the grill.

Lightly oil the grill, next preheat to medium-high.

Transfer the salmon fillets from the bag to a plate, pouring remaining marinade over the filet. Sprinkle with sea salt and black pepper, then place filets skin-side up on the grill for 2 minutes. Flip the salmon (skin-side down) and grill until cooked, about 6 minutes depending on the thickness of the filet.

Serve with brown rice or quinoa, a side salad, or sautéed veggies if desired

Coconut Curry Shrimp & Green Beans

2 pounds raw Shrimp

1 pound Green Beans, ends trimmed

1 (14 oz.) can Light Coconut Milk

2 Shallots, chopped

3 cloves Garlic, diced

4 teaspoons Curry Powder

1 teaspoon Paprika

2 tablespoons Extra Virgin Olive Oil

2 tablespoons Tapioca

3 cups cooked Brown Rice (optional)

Preheat a large skillet on medium-high heat. Add the oil and the green beans to the skillet and sauté for 3-4 minutes, stirring often, until the green beans just start to brown and soften slightly. Add the garlic and shallots and cook for another minute.

Turn the heat down to medium, then add the coconut milk, curry powder, paprika, and tapioca starch and whisk until well-combined. Add shrimp, cover and bring to a boil. Once the mixture is boiling, take off the lid and cook for another 5-8 minutes. It is done when the shrimp are opaque and cooked through.

Spicy Bacon Egg Salad

2 pieces nitrate-free turkey bacon, cooked and chopped

1/3 cup thinly sliced green onions

2 tablespoons plain non-fat Greek yogurt (nondairy yogurt recipe in back)

1 tablespoon mayo (or use another tablespoon Greek yogurt)

2 teaspoons Sriracha

1/4 teaspoon pepper

1/8 teaspoon sea salt

6 large hard-boiled eggs, peeled and chopped

Lettuce wraps, for serving

Stir together first 8 ingredients in medium bowl.

Portion and serve on lettuce wraps.

Cod with Spiced Red Lentils

1 cup red lentil

$\frac{1}{4}$ teaspoon ground turmeric

2 $\frac{1}{2}$ cups fish stock

2 tablespoons vegetable oil

1 ½ teaspoons cumin seeds

1 tablespoon grated ginger

½ teaspoon cayenne pepper

1 tablespoon lemon juice

2 tablespoons chopped fresh coriander

1 lb. cod fish fillet, skinned and cut into large chunks

Himalayan sea salt, to taste

Juice from 1 lemon

Put the lentils in a saucepan with the turmeric and stock. Bring to the boil, cover with a lid and simmer for 20-25 minutes, until the lentils are tender. Remove from the heat and add the salt.

Heat the oil in a small cast iron skillet. Add the cumin seeds and when they begin to pop, add the ginger and cayenne pepper. Stir-fry the spices for a few seconds, next pour in your lentils. Add the lemon juice and the coriander and stir them gently into the mixture. Transfer the mixture to an oven-proof 9-by-13 baking dish and Lay the pieces of cod on top of the lentils, bake for 30 minutes until the fish is flaky and tender.

Red Pepper and Lentil Bake

1 teaspoon olive oil

1 large onion, peeled and finely chopped

1 garlic clove, peeled and finely chopped

1/2 cup lentils

2 1/2 cups low-sodium, organic vegetable broth

4 red bell peppers, deseeded and chopped

1 large Granny Smith apple, peeled, cored, and chopped

2 teaspoons dried basil

1/4 cup white wine

14 ounces canned chopped tomatoes

1 ounce shredded cheddar cheese

1/3 ounce shredded parmesan cheese

Salt and pepper to taste

Preheat your oven to 350 degrees.

Heat the olive oil gently in a large saucepan, add onion and garlic, and cook until translucent.

Add the lentils and stir, next add your vegetable stock. Bring to a boil, then reduce heat and simmer for 25 minutes.

After it has cooked for 25 minutes. Add the peppers, basil, apple, white wine, and canned tomatoes and stir to combine.

Transfer the mixture to an oven-proof 9-by-13 baking dish and sprinkle cheese on top. Cook in oven for 30 minutes.

Loaded Turkey Stuffed-Twice Baked Sweet Potatoes

1 lb. ground turkey

1 can of black beans, rinsed and drained

2 large sweet potatoes

1/4 cup hot sauce

1 tablespoon coconut oil

1 yellow onion, diced

1 garlic clove, minced

2 teaspoons chipotle chili powder

1 teaspoon ground red pepper

1 teaspoon garlic powder

1 teaspoon onion powder

½ teaspoon paprika

Salt and pepper, to taste

Preheat your oven to 425 degrees.

Cut your sweet potatoes in half, lengthwise and put them facing cut side down on a cookie sheet. Put in the oven to cook for about 25-30 minutes depending how thick they are. You will know when they are done if they are easy to push on, on the skin side. If you pull them out early and the inside doesn't come out easily with a spoon, you'll need to cook them a bit longer.

While your sweet potatoes cook, put out a pot or skillet over medium-high heat. Add the coconut oil to the hot pan then add your garlic and onions to Sautee.

Once the onions are translucent, add the ground turkey and use a large spoon to break it up to help cook it a bit quicker.

When the turkey is half way done cooking, add the spices and your black beans. Let the turkey cook until no longer pink or until completely cooked through, take off heat.

Bring your sweet potatoes out of the oven and use a large spoon to scoop out the insides. Be careful to not go all the way to the skin or it may tear.

Add the sweet potatoes to your pan of turkey and mix to combine.

Now scoop out the new mixture and put into your sweet potato skins.

Place the loaded sweet potatoes back on the cookie sheet, face up, back into the oven and cook for 5-7 more minutes just to meld the flavors together and harden the top a bit.

Sweet Corn Chowder with Hot-Smoked Salmon

Ingredients

1 tablespoon non-dairy or non-soy butter

2 cups chopped onion

1 1/2 cups cubed peeled baking potato

3 cups fat-free, less-sodium chicken broth

1 1/2 cups fresh corn kernels

1 (15-ounce) can no-salt-added cream-style corn

1/4 teaspoon freshly ground black pepper

1/8 teaspoon ground red pepper

2 (4.5-ounce) packages hot-smoked salmon, flaked

4 teaspoons chopped fresh chives

Directions:

Melt butter in a large saucepan over medium-high heat. Add onion; sauté 4 minutes until soft. Add potato and broth; bring to a boil. Reduce heat, and simmer 10 minutes or until potato is tender. Add corn kernels and cream-style corn; cook 5 minutes. Stir in peppers. Ladle 1 1/4 cups chowder into each of 4 soup bowls. Divide salmon evenly among bowls. Garnish each serving with 1 teaspoon chives.

Quinoa & Tuna Salad

1 cup of cooked quinoa

2 cans albacore tuna, drained

1 can of petite baby sweet peas, drained and rinsed

2 roma tomatoes, chopped

½ cup red bell pepper, diced

¼ cup red onion, diced

1/2 c. mayonnaise

1 teaspoon of garlic, minced

1 t. onion powder

Plenty of salt and pepper to taste

It's so simple! Mix everything in a bowl and serve.

Fire Roasted tomato quinoa penne pasta with crispy chickpeas and zucchini

- 1 can fire roasted diced tomatoes, not drained
- 1 cup organic uncooked zucchini, diced
- 1 can (15 oz.) cooked chickpeas
- 2 tablespoon goats cheese, crumbles
- 2 cloves garlic, minced
- 2 tablespoon olive oil
- 8 oz. quinoa penne pasta
- Celtic sea salt and pepper to taste

Cook the quinoa pasta according to package, drain and set aside. Meanwhile in a large cast iron skillet, heat 1 tablespoon of olive oil and sauté zucchini, garlic and chickpeas over medium-high heat for about 12 minutes. After the chickpeas have cooked and become browned and crispy. Add the cooked pasta with zucchini, roasted tomatoes, and chickpeas. Mix well. Cook additional 5 minutes to allow and blend all the flavorings together. Season to taste and sprinkle goat cheese crumbles.

Mushroom-stuffed Omelet

I love eating breakfast for dinner. Having mushrooms, onions, and eggs are a great way to boost selenium levels. Here is a quick recipe that is both filling and super easy to whip up.

Ingredients:

4 organic or cage free eggs

3 medium-sized mushrooms, diced

½ tablespoon coconut oil or ½ tablespoon of avocado oil

A teaspoon of dairy free and soy free butter

Salt and pepper to taste

Directions:

In a cast iron skillet add a ½ tablespoon of coconut oil or avocado oil and sauté the mushrooms till they are golden brown. While mushrooms are browning.

Whisk eggs with seasonings in a bowl. After the mushrooms have browned. Add the teaspoon of butter. Stir the butter around the pan so it can get completely coated and mixed with the mushrooms.

Add the egg mixture, it will take about 1 minute for the egg to set and then flip over. Heat for another 30 seconds, then remove from pan. Place on a plate.

Smoked Turkey, tomato & brown Rice Bake

1 tablespoon extra-virgin olive oil

1 cup thinly sliced celery

½ cup onion, diced

1 28-ounce can diced tomatoes

1 cup low-fat, no-salt-added cottage cheese

1 cup instant brown rice

6 ounces smoked turkey breast

1/4 cup water

1 teaspoon freshly ground pepper, or to taste

1 cup goat cheese

Heat oil in a cast iron skillet over medium-high heat. Cook celery and onion, stirring frequently, until beginning to soften, 2 to 3 minutes. Transfer the mixture to an oven-proof 9-by-13 baking dish and sprinkle cheese on top. Cook in oven for 15 minutes. Bake, uncovered, until most of the liquid has evaporated. Spread cheese on top. Broil until the cheese is bubbling, 2 to 3 minutes.

Savory Chicken Casserole

2 c cooked shredded chicken

1.5 c butternut squash, peeled and cubed

1/2 c coconut cream (skimmed off of the top of a can of coconut milk)

2 Tbsp. coconut oil, melted

1 cup green peas

1 TBSP apple cider vinegar

1 tsp sea salt

1 tsp garlic powder

1/2 tsp black pepper

1/2 tsp oregano

1/2 tsp thyme

1/2 tsp onion powder

Place your butternut squash in a large pot of boiling water for approximately 40 minutes. Remove butternut squash from pot using a strainer and place in a large bowl. Using a potato masher, mash butternut squash to a smooth, but leave a somewhat chunky texture. Add apple cider vinegar, sea salt, garlic powder, black pepper, oregano, thyme and onion powder to the mashed butternut squash and mix to combine. Add the coconut cream and oil, mixing to combine. Stir in coconut oil, coconut cream, shredded chicken and green peas. Transfer the mixture to an oven-proof 9-by-13 baking dish. Cook for approximately 8-10 minutes on medium heat.

Slow Cooker Quinoa, Chicken and Butternut Squash Soup

1 medium butternut squash, peeled and cubed

14 oz. can coconut milk, full fat

2 cups water

2 tbsp. raw honey or maple syrup

1 tbsp. red curry paste

1 inch ginger, peeled & grated

1 garlic clove, crushed

1 1/2 tsp salt

1.5 lbs. chicken breast

2 cups quinoa, cooked

2 large red bell peppers, thinly sliced

1/4 cup cilantro, chopped

1/2 lime, juice of

In a large slow cooker, add squash, coconut milk, water, honey, curry paste, ginger, garlic, salt, lime leaves and chicken. Cover and cook on Low for 8 hours or on High for 4 hours. Remove chicken and shred using two forks. Using immersion blender, blend soup until smooth. Add chicken, quinoa, bell peppers, cilantro and lime juice. Stir and enjoy!

Turkey Chili

2 lbs. 99% fat-free ground turkey

1 yellow onion, diced

5 cloves garlic, minced

1 Tbsp. olive oil

1 (28 oz.) can crushed tomatoes, no-salt added

1 (15 oz.) can petite diced tomatoes, no-salt added

3 Tbsp. tomato paste

½ tsp. hot sauce

1 (15 oz.) can kidney beans, no-salt added, drained and rinsed

1 red bell pepper, chopped

1 green bell pepper, chopped

2 jalapenos, chopped

1¼ tsp. sea salt

Pinch of pepper

3 Tbsp. chili powder

2 tsp. oregano

⅛ Tsp. cayenne pepper

Drizzle olive oil in a large pot and sauté onion and garlic until fragrant, about 3 minutes. Add ground turkey and cook until crumbled and brown, draining excess liquid as necessary. Add all the rest of the ingredients and cook on medium/low heat for about an hour. Enjoy!

Hawaiian Crockpot Chicken

2 large chicken breast

1/3 cup coconut aminos

1/2 cup coconut sugar

10 oz can pineapple rings

1 green bell pepper, deseeded and large chopped

Place chicken in the bottom of your crockpot. Mix coconut aminos and coconut sugar together then pour over chicken. Place pineapple rings and bell pepper around the chicken. .Cook for 3-4 hours on high or 6-8 on low. When done, dice chicken into bite-sized pieces and serve. This would be fantastic with ½ cup of brown rice and ½ cup of cooker green beans.

"Creamy" Chicken Tomato Soup Slow Cooker

4 frozen skinless boneless chicken breast

Garlic salt to taste

2 tablespoons Italian Seasoning

1 tablespoon dried basil

1 clove garlic

1 14 oz. can of coconut milk (full fat)

1 14 oz. can diced tomatoes and juice

1 cup of chicken broth

Sea Salt and pepper to taste

Put all the above ingredients into the crock-pot, cook for 9 hours on low. After 9 hours take two forks and shred the chicken, set the crock-pot on warm till ready to serve. For a creamier soup, before adding back the shredded chicken. Blend some of the soup and put it back in the slow cooker. You can this in batches in a regular blend but remember it's hot or use an immersion hand held blender.

Snacks, Drinks and Tonic's

Mayo

1 large egg

2 tablespoon mustard

1.5 cups of olive oil

1 teaspoon of vinegar

2 teaspoons of lemon juice

½ teaspoon of Himalayans sea salt

Combine everything in a 32 oz mason jar. Using an immense hand held blender blend until smooth. If you don't have a immersion blender.

In a blender, blend the egg and mustard until well blended. Slowly drizzle in the olive oil and continue until it becomes thick and emulsified. Add the vinegar and lemon juice. Slow add your salt and adjust the taste if needed.

Dark Chocolate coconut apricot bites

5 dried Apricots

1/2 ounce dark chocolate

Sprinkle some coarse Celtic sea salt and shredded coconut

Lay a piece of parchment paper on a plate. Heat dark chocolate in a small bowl in the microwave at 20 second intervals. Stir often and heat until JUST melted (chocolate burns easily in the microwave). Dip 1/2 apricot in the chocolate, put on plate, and dust with salt. Refrigerate for 1/2 hour and serve.

No-bake oatmeal bites

1 cup dry quick oats

2/3 cup coconut flakes

1/2 cup almond butter

1/2 cup dark chocolate chips

1/3 cup raw honey

1 tsp vanilla

Directions: Mix all ingredients, form into 1 inch balls. Place balls in refrigerator and snack away.

Fried Chickpeas

2 teaspoons smoked paprika

1 teaspoon cayenne pepper

6 tablespoons extra-virgin olive oil

2 15-oz. cans chickpeas, rinsed, drained, patted very dry

Kosher salt

2 teaspoons finely grated lime zest

Combine paprika and cayenne in a small bowl and set aside.

Heat oil in a cast iron skillet over medium-high heat. Working in 2 batches, add chickpeas to skillet and sauté, stirring frequently, until golden and crispy, 15-20 minutes. Using a slotted spoon, transfer chickpeas to paper towels to get excess oil off. Transfer to a bowl. Sprinkle paprika mixture over; toss to coat. Season to taste with salt. Toss with lime zest and serve. You can eat this over a bowl of brown rice or quinoa.

Spicy pumpkin seeds

Dash of Himalayan sea salt

1 teaspoon of coconut oil

¼ teaspoon of smoked paprika

¼ teaspoon of garlic powder

1/8 teaspoon of chili powder

1 cup of raw pumpkin seeds

Melt coconut oil. Mix everything with the seeds in a bowl. Lay seeds on a baking dish. Roast for 20 minutes tossing after 10. Make sure they don't become overly brown. That means the inside of the seed is burning.

Skin-tactic Water

8 glasses water

1 tsp grated ginger root (optional)

1 medium-sized cucumber, peeled and cut into slices

1 medium-sized lemon cut into slices

12 fresh mint leaves

Direction:

Mix all the ingredients in a large pitcher, leave them overnight. Drink all the next day. Voila!

Lemon, Ginger and Turmeric tea

This is an amazing morning go-to drink. It's healing, energizing, and hydrating. Turmeric is an antioxidant, cancer preventive, anti-inflammatory and aids in liver protection. Lemon does a fabulous job with alkalinizing the body, aid in digestion and boost your immune system. Ginger is anti-inflammatory, boost your immune system, lowers blood sugar, lowers cholesterol levels, cancer fighter, improve brain function, cold and flu prevention, and improves heart health. Gloves reduces inflammation, antiviral and anti-bacterial properties, improves digestion, aids in a sore throat, natural pain killer, helps with insomnia and aids in healthier teeth and gums. Cayenne pepper pain reliever, appetite suppressant, reduces blood sugar levels, helps remove toxins from the blood and improves blood circulation.

Word of caution. Pregnant women are advised to control consumption since it could stimulate the uterus.

1 whole lemon, sliced

1 tablespoon ginger, minced

2 cloves

1/8 teaspoon turmeric

2 1/2 cups boiling water

Pinch of cayenne

Place the lemon slices, ginger, cloves, and turmeric in a teapot. Pour your boiling water in your teapot. Allow to steep for 30 minutes. Strain over your cup. Just before serving add a dash of cayenne pepper. If you feel a sore throat coming on add 2 teaspoons of raw honey. Honey is a natural cough suppressant, antibacterial properties and will help reduce swelling and discomfort. If you want it creamy you can always add coconut milk or almond milk.

Repeat for 12 cookies per sheet (will take 6 cookie sheets for whole recipe).

Bake for 5 minutes. Watch carefully as they burn quickly. Remove from oven and let sit on baking sheet for at least 2 minutes (do not try to remove before then).Remove from baking sheet using a spatula and let cool completely on a wire rack. Will keep for several days on counter in an airtight container.

Dairy-free Coconut Yogurt

2-14 oz. cans coconut milk

2 teaspoons agar agar flakes or 2 tablespoons tapioca starch

4 probiotic capsules

2 tablespoons raw sugar or grade B maple syrup, (optional)

Warm you oven and make sure you jars are sterilized. Warm your oven for about 5 minutes until it reaches 100 F, then turn off the heat.

Shake the can of coconut milk 1st before pouring into a sauce pan. Next add your thickener. If you're using agar agar, sprinkle 1 teaspoon of the agar agar flakes into the pot over the coconut milk- but don't stir. If you are using the tapioca starch, scoop out roughly 1/3 cup of the coconut milk and whisk the starch in the milk. Make sure it is completely dissolved then add it back to the sauce pan.

Continue to Heat the coconut milk over the heat until it begins to simmer. Whisk the milk and turn it down on low. Continue cooking on low, whisking occasionally for an additional 10 minutes. Until the agar agar is full dissolved or the tapioca starch has thickened the milk.

Cool your milk until it reaches the temperature of 100 F. Next twist open your probiotic capsules and pour it into your milk. Whisk to combine. Add your agar or syrup if you desire and whisk that in.

Pour into jars, seal the lids on them and allow the yogurt to sit for 12-24 hours at 110 F in the oven or a dehydrator without disrupting. After it has completed its cycle, place in the fridge to chill for no less than 6 hours. The yogurt will become thicker as it sits and chills. If you find the mixture to have separated and is yellowish of color, don't be alarmed, just give it a good stir to combine again. This coconut yogurt will last up to 2 weeks in the fridge.

If the yogurt develops a pink or grey discoloration on its surface that means it has been contaminated with bad bacteria. Throw it away and do not eat it!

If you want a super thick Greek style yogurt. The night before place your canned coconut milk in the fridge. Don't not shake. In the morning when you open it, scoop out the thick hardened top layer part of the cream. Discard the "liquidy" coconut water underneath it.

Non-dairy buttermilk

Place 1 tablespoon lemon juice, lime juice, apple cider vinegar, or white vinegar in a measuring cup.

Add enough non-dairy milk (of your choosing) until it reaches the 1-cup line; stir with a fork or whisk.

Allow mixture to rest for 5-10 minutes.

Voila, you have your Non-dairy buttermilk!

Alcohol

I would love to say that we shouldn't drink at all during our 21 day reboot but let's face it that isn't realistic. So the trick is to choose wisely. Wine is full of flavonoids and antioxidants. If you can find a wine that is organic or no added sulfites that would be perfect. Wine isn't as hard on the liver as hard alcohol. The worst thing to sip on is brewed beer, tequila and rum. It causes blood sugar imbalances and bloating. **Vodka** is the simplest of spirits and consists almost entirely of water and ethanol. It's distilled many times to a very high proof, removing almost all impurities, and then watered down to desired strength. Since just about all impurities are removed, it can be made from just about anything. All vodka is gluten-free unless it is a "flavored vodka" where someone adds a gluten-containing ingredient.

Homemade deodorant

I've been making my own deodorant for years. It all started when I came across an article on the internet about how aluminum-based antiperspirants may increase the risk for breast cancer, Alzheimer's Disease & Kidney Disease (Scientists noticed that dialysis patients who had these high aluminum levels were more likely to develop dementia too.) Our bodies are supposed to sweat. Sweat isn't inherently stinky either. In fact, it's nearly odorless. The stench comes from bacteria that break down from one of two types of sweat on your skin. Deodorant advertisers have done a pretty neat job of convincing us that we're disgustingly smelly people who in fact need to be refined and save our stinky self's by their products. We've been wonderfully brain washed into thinking sweating is a bad thing. Sweating from the heat, sweating from exercise and sweating from stress are all different, chemically speaking. Stress sweat smells the worst. That's because smelly sweat is only produced by one of the two types of sweat glands called the apocrine glands, which are usually in areas with lots of hair, like our armpits, the groin area and scalp. The odor is the result of the bacteria that break down the sweat once it's released onto your skin. Fun fact: While women have more sweat glands than men, men's sweat glands produce more sweat.

Ingredients

1/2 c. baking soda

1/2 c. arrowroot powder or ½ cup of cornstarch

5 tbsp. unrefined virgin coconut oil

10 drops of grapefruit essential oil or lavender essential oil

You can pick your favorite scent. I like lavender or grapefruit.

Directions

Mix baking soda and arrowroot together.

Melt your coconut oil in the microwave in a microwave safe bowl.

Mix all ingredients the baking soda and arrowroot powder with the oil, Pour into clean small Mason jar, add your essential oil to the Mason jar, close with the lid. Give it a good shake to combine the essential oil with the other mixture. By doing it this way. You can still use that bowl to eat with. Once you mix that essential oil in the bowl, it can only be used for the purpose of making your deodorant. Everything you've used is edible except the essential oils.

This will take roughly 24 hours to set. It will thicken up. I use my finger to scrape what I need and scoop it across my underarm.

Homemade all natural shampoo

2/3 cup of castile soap

Two teaspoons of almond or olive oil

10 drops of your favorite food grade essential oil

½ cup of coconut milk

Mix all the ingredients in a bottle. Use when needed.

Did you know that your teeth are living and spongy. The foods we eat, the commercial toothpastes, medications and chemicals from drinks all can suck out the minerals from the teeth causing weakened enamel and leaving us more susceptible to decay and breakdown. I was on a new mission to keep my teeth healthy by using the absolute necessary and needed trace minerals to maintain the upmost dental health plus find a solution that wasn't abrasive, while gently polishing them, and detoxifies while it refreshes. Is there such a thing? I did know that my long history with Mr. Store bought toothpaste were over. Bentonite clay does its work drawing toxins out of the mouth, it leaves behind minerals that are nourishing for the teeth. Try my homemade toothpaste.

Natural Tooth Paste Recipe

Natural Peppermint Toothpaste

1/2 cup coconut oil

3 Tablespoons of baking soda

15 drops of peppermint food grade essential oil

Melt to soften the coconut oil. Mix in other ingredients and stir well. Place your mixture into small glass jar. Allow it to cool completely. When ready to use just dip toothbrush in and scrape small amount onto bristles.

Homemade Coconut Oil Toothpaste Recipe

6 tbsp. coconut oil

6 tbsp. baking soda

15-20 drops of a food grade essential oil (peppermint, cinnamon, grapefruit or lemon taste great)

Melt to soften the coconut oil. Mix in other ingredients and stir well. Place your mixture into small glass jar. Allow it to cool completely. When ready to use just dip toothbrush in and scrape small amount onto bristles.

Homemade Tooth Powder Recipe

Ingredients

- 4 tablespoons Bentonite clay
- 2 teaspoons baking soda
- 1 ½ teaspoons finely ground unrefined sea salt
- ½ teaspoons clove powder
- 1 teaspoon ground Ceylon cinnamon
- 5-10 drops of peppermint essential oil
- ¾ teaspoons activated charcoal –

Directions

Using a stainless steel or plastic spoon, mix all ingredients in a clean glass jar. To use, add a little to a wet toothbrush and brush as normal.

Natural Peppermint Toothpaste

1/2 cup coconut oil

3 Tablespoons of baking soda

15 drops of peppermint food grade essential oil

Melt to soften the coconut oil. Mix in other ingredients and stir well. Place your mixture into small glass jar. Allow it to cool completely. When ready to use just dip toothbrush in and scrape small amount onto bristles.

Body Butter

- 4 oz. Shea butter
- 1 oz. coconut oil
- 1 oz. jojoba oil
- 6 drops cypress essential oil
- 4 drops cinnamon essential oil
- 6 drops wild orange essential oil
- 3 drops of pure vanilla extract
- 1 teaspoon of Vitamin E oil

In a double boiler over simmering water completely melt your shea butter. Remove from heat and add your coconut oil and jojoba oil. Blend together gently until completely mixed. Place the double boiler into an ice bath, make sure to not get any water into the mixture. Continue to mix until it begins to turn opaque. Lastly add your essential oils/extract/and antioxidant while stirring. I prefer to use a hand mixer to whip the mixture gently to where it will give it a soufflé-like texture.

After the mixture has cooled to room temperature transfer the body butter to a mason jar with a sealable lid using the spatula to avoid wasting any of the body butter. Seal the jar with your lid and allow it to sit overnight. Make sure to label and date your body butter's lid.

Homemade "Vaseline"

Ingredients

- 1/4 cup coconut oil

1/8 cup olive oil

2 tablespoons beeswax

2 drops peppermint essential oil (optional or your favorite smell)

Over medium heat you want to melt the coconut oil and beeswax to combine. After its melted remove from the heat, pour in the EVOO and mix the ingredients together. Allow it to cool but you want it still pour-able so you can pour the mixture into a mason jar and add your essential oil which is optional. This homemade Vaseline will keep fresh on the counter for up to a year.

DIY Skin Smoother Detox Bath

2 cups Epsom salt

2 cups baking soda

2 cups sea salt

1 cup vinegar

¼ cup of organic coconut oil (this will melt in the hot bath)

Directions: combine the dry ingredients, store in a closed container. When you are ready to take a bath add 1 cup of dry ingredients, 1 cup of vinegar and ¼ cup of coconut oil. (Kids can use up to a 1/2 cup of the mixture). Bathe 3 times weekly, soaking for at least 12 minutes.

Bathroom Mold disinfecting spray

You don't have to grab bleach to get rid of mold in your bathroom. This 3 combo all natural mixture will do the trick. I will spray the areas in my bathroom and leave it on for 10 minutes and wipe the moldy areas away. Vodka might be a little bit pricey but you won't be breathing in toxic chemicals or having to worry about your skin absorbing a list of toxic chemicals. Vinegar is naturally antimicrobial, tea tree is natural fungicide which can eliminate any mold or mildew problems and kills black mold spores! Don't forget to label your spray bottle with a black permanent marker.

1 cup of white vinegar

1 cup of vodka

20 drops of tea tree oil

No diluting this combo. Mix well in a spray bottle and label it bathroom mold killer. Spray onto hard surfaces where mold and mildew are growing and let this amazing combo go to work. You'll still have to scrub a bit, but with repeated use this all-natural cleaner will kill the fungus and help to prevent future growth. Shake each time before use. Don't forget to label your spray bottle with a black permanent marker.

Easy Floor cleaner

1 cup of white vinegar

1 tablespoon of Sal Suds

1 cup of baking soda

2 gallons of very warm water

Mix all in a bucket and enjoy mopping your floors with a nontoxic cleaner.

Awareness has magic!

Don't exhaust yourself trying to figure out why you're sick. Start looking for the root. Pull back the curtain and let your body know that you are listening. You see the enemy is scheming against you. He wants you to be unhappy, jealous and envious.

You know that healthy habits make sense, but did you ever stop to think why you practice them?

I've heard women, in particular, say this a lot lately. They say, "Why can't I look like that?!" I will never look like that!"

Why do we mentally sabotage ourselves? Let's get something clear. You are unique. You are not meant to be me & I am not meant to be you. We are on this planet as individuals, each of us has a unique finger print that can't and won't ever be duplicated with any other human being. Ever! So why do you mentally sabotage your mindset with self-doubt and in return it starts a domino effect on your health? You are telling your subconscious without even realizing it that you are not made for greater things. You are telling your subconscious that you cannot be sexy, be brilliant and be fantastic. Be happy in your skin.

Everywhere you look — on every billboard, on every social media channel — it seems that there are beautiful, scantily clad women. So it is pushed down our throats that beauty starts from the outside but actually its starts on the inside and radiates outward.

Here's the thing: if you treat your body like it's your worst enemy – or not take ownership of your physical well-being – you are repelling good health. You're keeping yourself from being the best you can be in your life, because you dislike your body so much.

You're basically saying, "I dislike good health. I want to be rid of it."

Well, wish granted!

Good nutrition is an important part of leading a healthy lifestyle.

You're meant to make a difference in this world; that's why you're here. But you must believe you're meant for greater things, so you can actually enter a place of mental stability, and eventually, a place of fantastic health. Don't take yourself out of the game by ignoring your bad relationship with your health.

Common ways that we keep Ourselves Sick. Luckily, you can fix them.

Improve your relationship with your health

When you decide to improve your relationship with your health, be prepared for people to question and criticize you. Change can be a very difficult thing for many of us to handle. You have the mindset, to step out on faith to get the perfect health that you really wish to have. It could be from grabbing that apple instead of those chips, walking 10 minutes per day, or reading a self-help book.

Take Action: Let yourself out of that unhealthy, fast-food, over processed and artificially filled food habit because it's ruining your life. The only way to create a different outcome is to allow yourself to forgive what's happened in the past. The past does not have to be your future. You are 100% capable of changing your future health story, so do it.

You never step outside your box.

"I can't afford eat better."

"I don't want to spend the money on a new diet book."

"I wish, someone would just give me the magic pill for my ideal body!"

"I don't want to purchase another program that isn't going to work."

Does any of this sound familiar? The more you focus on what you don't have, the less likely it is that you'll ever have it.

Take Action: Focus on what you do have right now. Express gratitude for literally being alive. Now, you have to create a strategy to have what you really want. Set a goal, writing down realistic goals and make yourself a deadline. Take steps to get there. (And don't quit if it doesn't work the very first try.)

Or… you can keep focusing on what you lack. Call me in a year and tell me how that's working out for you.

You think health is something you're granted with, rather than invest.

You want your health to work for you, so you have to think of everything you eat as an investment. Will eating that cheeseburger build or create that healthy body? Probably not.

Will investing in self-improvement books or a mentorship program? Perhaps, if you do the work and commit to changing old habits.

Take Action: When you're about to improve your health, think carefully about why you're about to modify your life with. If that item, service or experience is worth it. Then ask yourself:

Will it feel like a good investment in 90 days, 6 months, or even a year?

Will it help you create a healthier you?

Will it help create a happier you?

Will this change bring you immense joy and memories that will last forever?

Will you grow as a result?

Investing in your health will have a high return, personally and professionally. Don't go foolishly looking for cheap thrills and expect to be in better state of health this time next year. Believe that you're worthy of investing in yourself and believe you'll have a return.

You can reduce your exposure to them by eating organic foods, making your own cleaning chemicals and using alternative pest control methods.

My story

After being diagnosed with hypothyroidism over 25 years ago. I knew there was something more than just being labeled with a medical condition. There wasn't a lot of information on how to heal myself.

I felt as if I had lost control over my body and my mental health as well. It seems that I had experienced every symptom from lack of energy, anxiety, weight gain, scary heart palpitations and brain fog. I couldn't sleep and where the hell had my eye brows gone? My hair loss was thinning, I was always constipated, my blood pressure started to increase, my fingertips would get cold and numb just out of the blue, my emotions were all over the place, I was on an emotional roller coaster. I had aches and pains that it seemed hard to explain to my doctor and my doctor thought it was all in my head. My doctor wanted to give me thyroid medication plus antidepressants. I was not depressed. The simplest tasks seemed like the hardest on some days. I really didn't realize or understand the whole life impact that my "new" condition, because as I started investigating I realized that all the wide ranging symptoms of hypothyroidism were being brushed off by my doctor at the time as being part of everyday life, stress or getting older.

It seemed no matter what diet I tried, I couldn't lose the weight. No matter what exercise I tried, I couldn't shed the weight. What I was missing and what I didn't figure out until much later is that there were many things at play with my health and weight loss battle. The thyroid medication that I was taking was synthetic T4. I needed my T3 to be converted as well. See, my T3 was my energy hormone and I suffered from this horrible imbalance of my T4 not converting to T3 which lead to my adrenal fatigue. My system was so over worked, I had a lack of nutrients and my body was severely imbalanced. The adrenal fatigue put my body in a battle and my cortisol levels were out of this world! Cortisol added fat around my mid-section. So, the harder I exercised, the more "cortisol"-fat added to my stomach. Then let's mention the leaky gut. My gut played a vital role in my autoimmunity. 95% of all thyroid diseases are autoimmune. Most often this is undiagnosed. I needed to get my gut fixed. The only way I was going to start to put my Hashimoto's in remission is to start working on my gut. The 70% of my immune system is manufactured in my gut. Like an onion, I started to work on each layer that needed to be addressed, peeling it back, layer by layer. Did I have food sensitives? Many people have food sensitives continue to eat these foods that causes a leaky gut, candida and ph imbalances. Gluten, dairy, soy, eggs and processed foods are just to name a few. Also, no matter how much I worked on my foods and exercise. It wasn't going do me any good if I continued to use household cleaners, aluminum under arm deodorants and fluoride toothpastes. The list can go on and one. I needed to start reading labels and not allow these toxins on my body. I was fighting an uphill battle for my life. I started by the elimination process. Uncovered what foods bothered me, fixed my gut, slowed down my exercise and had my doctor help me tweak my medication. I started reading food labels, if it was artificial or made in a lab I avoided it. If I couldn't eat it, I didn't put it on my body. I avoided all environmental toxins like the plague. I added vital vitamins and minerals that my body was missing and probiotics. This wasn't a "diet" it was a lifestyle change. A complete overhaul of my life in every aspect.

<u>I had to start listening to my body, and not one of those a dietary theories. I couldn't force foods that didn't agree with me on myself because someone else thought they were healthy. Dietary theories are meant to</u>

be a starting point, your body will give you further directions.

After being diagnosis, I was relieved and excited to finally have an answer, some kind of answer, to what was going on with my body but soon I was disappointed again only to find out that the thyroid medications that I thought was going bring you back to myself only fixed a few of my symptoms and I was still having to deal with a dozen more remaining issues. I was so tired of hearing that it was all in my head. I wanted to scream to the world and let everyone know that my quality of life had drastically been affected and there has to be answers.

Somewhere, Someone, Anyone at this point, hello? Help me, I feel like I am drowning, slowly dying and the world just keeps turning. Why isn't anyone listening to me?

My quality of life has been affected.

Every Cell in my body responds to the foods that I eat, the products that I put on my body to the house hold chemicals that I purchase for my home. All of these things have a direct impact on my hormones and in return my hormones have a direct impact on every major system in my body. Not to mention that my body was lacking certain nutrients that heavily influence the function of every cell in my body.

The foods that I consume, oh, the foods I consume.

I've learned in my journey that organic, whole, nutrient rich food is medicine. I really can't say it any simpler than that. There is a major disconnect between what we believe to be healthy foods and what research tells us is healthy. In fact, many of the health foods today that people go out of their way to eat daily are extremely thyroid suppressive.

I started to become my very own health investigator. I started researching what I need to do to start addressing what the root cause that lead to me to this point in my life. I certainly wouldn't take Motrin if I got a pebble stuck in my shoe? So, why am I going to take this new medication for my thyroid if I didn't understand how I got here?

As I began researching I soon discovered that hypothyroidism does has a root issue. I often ignored all the underlying causes of my hypothyroidism. What was I looking for? Like an onion, I needed to see it layer by layer. I started to do a little pruning of my branches, I wanted to be healthy again. My thyroid was being influenced by many so many different things.

You see, the main problem with hypothyroidism is that it's a very tricky condition and complicated disorder to manage. There is no one size fits all program when you are dealing with hypothyroidism.

Around 20 million Americans and 250 million people worldwide will be affected by low thyroid function or hypothyroidism. One in 8 women will struggle with a thyroid problem in her lifetime, and up to 90% of all thyroid problems are autoimmune in nature, the most common of which is Hashimoto's. As diseases go, you would think that it would be a cinch to diagnose and pretty straightforward to treat. Many people don't know that hypothyroidism is an autoimmune disease and the reason why most doctors don't mention is because it's simple: it doesn't affect their treatment plan. Traditional medicine treats autoimmune disorders with steroids and other methods that suppress the immune system. The number of people suffering from hypothyroidism continues to rise each year. Levothyroxine is the 4th highest selling drug in the U.S. THE 4TH HIGHEST SELLING DRUG!

Every Cell in your body responds to your thyroid hormones. These hormones have a direct impact on every major system in your body.

As consumers we put our trust in the research and development of scientific studies, The FDA and The CDC. Drug store chains have quota's to meet and even some of our Doctors get yearly bonus's. Little do we do that behind closed doors corporations often pay scientists and these companies to support their product for profit. Some Politicians seem to have a revolving door between the private and public sector. The synthetic chemicals we face every day that is in our food, our water, and the air that we breathe.

Did you know that products we use every day may contain toxic chemicals and has been linked to women's health issues? They are hidden endocrine disruptors and are very tricky chemicals that play havoc on our bodies. "We are all routinely exposed to endocrine disruptors, and this has the potential to significantly harm the health of our youth," said Renee Sharp, EWG's director of research. "It's important to do what we can to avoid them, but at the same time we can't shop our way out of the problem. We need to have a real chemical policy reform. "The longer the length of ingredients on your food or body product labels means how much more unhealthy it is for you to consume or place on your body. When an item contains a host of ingredients that most likely you can't even pronounce or remember to spell you can bet your lucky dollar that the natural nutrients are long gone. These highly processed frank n foods or body products are very difficult for the body to break down and some of the chemicals will become stored in your body. Your body doesn't know how to process it, so it gets stored.

No wonder our bodies are completely bombarded and overwhelmed with the constant exposed to toxic chemicals through the air that we breathe, the water we drink, the foods we eat, and the personal care products and cleaning products we use.

After being diagnosed with hypothyroidism over 25 years ago. I knew there was something more than just being labeled with this medical condition. There certainly wasn't a whole lot of information on how to heal myself. Continuing my research I began to understand that there really isn't a one size fits all diet for everyone who is has been diagnosed with Hypothyroidism but there are certain ways you can eat that will certainly help begin the healing process. Diet alone isn't enough to help your body start fighting this battle that is raging in your body. The food you eat is your first line of defense against hypothyroidism. You must start addressing other areas in your life.

This was a lifestyle change that I needed to pursue not another fade diet.

My new purpose is to empower people to embrace who they are, to add value to their life, to inspire them and to connect with those who are struggling with hypothyroidism. You need to realize that you have to invest in your health. You are worth investing money into yourself and take charge of your health. Will it "hurt" a little? Ha, you bet, but it will change your life.

I wish somebody had given me a step-by-step road-map back when I was first diagnosed with hypothyroidism. The solutions in this book has helped so many people. I've done my best to pull from all their expertise, as well as my own knowledge and clinical experience. I want to make it easy for you to find the answers quickly, all in the one place, because I'm all too familiar with that awful side effects of hypothyroidism. I certainly don't want you to have to spend years finding solutions, like I did. I also want you to understand that there isn't an easy "one pill" solution, but the "one pill" approach that our current medical system is using is NOT WORKING because the underlying cause for hypothyroidism is not being addressed.

It's been many years since I started on this journey of discovery. I've written many articles, a ton of blogging on my website Thehypothyroidismchick.com and published 6 books. My goal is to educate those who are on a similar path as mine with hypothyroidism. Lately, there's been something very deep nudging at my very core screaming to come out. I finally decided to let it seep out of my fingertips into this book. When I began writing about hypothyroidism, I knew it was an uncharted territory. My mindset was to search the truth, share my experiences and write compelling articles. The more I write, the more polished I become to develop my palate and skill-set. I have found something that I deeply care about and its worth every-bit of cherishing.

I write from the heart and share my truth.

I've realized that there will always be people who will always be a follower and never a leader when it comes to their health or their life in general. You must analyze your own truths and never from someone else's perceptive, always be your own life advocate and form your own truths with your own ideas of what is going to work in your life.

What I express in my blogs, books and articles are purely my views and opinions from the research and readings that I've done. I do not claim to have the absolute entire truth; this is simply what I have concluded at this moment in my life.

As each passing day goes, I continue to learn. As each passing day goes, I continue to grow.

We all have our very own skills and talents that we have to offer the world. I encourage you to find yours.

Let's get on thing straight.

I'm not trying to sell your health. I am trying to open your eyes and give you a purpose to start being healthy.

There is no such thing as something for nothing. So many people don't listen to their bodies. If you are constantly putting the wrong gas in your car is will start to eventually break down. Your body is the same way. One of the most common failure is the habit of quitting. Don't allow this type of failure of defeat to trick you into quitting. You are worth great health. You have the abundance of good health within your reach.

Being healthy is a state of mind. When you start to realize that the food you eat, the products you use and the way you live all talk to your DNA. Once you realize that you have a choice to change and you want to change you will change. You will start to read labels, you will think about what you're eating, how it was made and will it benefit your body.

Impossible? No! Not at all.

Being healthy does come from those with a healthy conscious. You and you alone must decide whether or not good health is important. Is good health worth the effort? You see we are wiping ourselves out. It seems with all the bad choices we are ultimately preparing ourselves for our own final destruction's. We often do choose badly but it's our choice to do so. The diet industry is a load of bullshit. Eat less, exercise more doesn't work. None of us should be on the same eating plan. What I mean by this is, each of us are unique. I may be allergic to eggs or dairy or gluten whereas someone else isn't. I may be need to take more vitamin b or vitamin d where your body is adequately great. I may need to eat more potassium rich foods where your body could have a potassium abundance. Working with a Knowledgeable Health Practitioner will do the proper blood work and screenings to see what exactly your body needs.

The main reason why you should work with a knowledgeable health practitioner is its patient-centered medical healing at its best. Unfortunately when it comes to hypothyroidism there isn't a one size fits all approach to dealing with it and often times you are left still searching for the answers to your symptoms when all you want is your zest for life back. A knowledgeable health practitioner will care for you as an individual as they won't look at your body as a whole they will treat each individual body symptom, imbalance and dysfunction. They certainly move from the confusion of the "one size fits all treatment" approach that we know isn't working to the one that will cater to what your body needs. Let's not forget that each of us are a unique case and unless you get a proper thorough clinical evaluation, trying to figure what medical advise you need online is dubious at best.

Imagine your body is one piece of machinery. Your entire body works together and if one area is affected it's like a domino effect on the other areas. It puts a strain on the other areas and they have to work harder to pull the weight of that area that not working like it should. So, start working on reducing your body's total load. Your health condition has a root cause. Once you start addressing the root of your problems is when your body can start healing itself. Your body is an awesome design but there is a complex balance between everything. It's a domino effect. Four things you must start doing immediately is getting your immune system in check, fixing your unhealthy gut, change your mindset and decrease your inflammation. Inflammation disrupts the production and regulatory mechanisms of hormones. Remember what I've already said: Sometimes we have to do a little pruning of the branches, in order for the tree to be healthy again.

Why? We are all different.

Break that cycle today, start eating to cater to your thyroid and replenish your life. Knowledge is power, educate yourself and find the answer to your health care needs. Wisdom is a wonderful thing to seek. I hope this book will teach and encourage you to take leaps in your life to educate yourself for a happier & healthier life.

You have the power to make a difference in your life. You've always had the power. No one can force you to become more aware of what you put on your body and what you put in your body. What you eat is just as important as what you put on your body. Adjusting your life, reading labels and catering to your specific health needs isn't easy but it will benefit you in the long run. This is one of the smartest decisions that you can make. Not only will you start to look and feel better but think of the medical cost that you could be saving your future self.

A full thyroid panel for hypothyroidism should at least include these key thyroid lab tests:

TSH

Free T4

Free T3

Reverse T3

Thyroid Peroxidase Antibodies

Thyroglobulin Antibodies

Listen TSH alone does not give a full picture of thyroid health.

Normal Ranges for you blood work

TSH- (range .034 - 4.82)

Free- T4 (range 0.59 - 1.17)

Total -T4 (range 4.5 - 12.0)

Total- T3 (range 71 - 180)

1. TSH (Thyroid Stimulating Hormone) TSH – This is a pituitary hormone that responds to low/high amounts of circulating thyroid hormone. In advanced cases of Hashimoto's and primary hypothyroidism, this lab test will be elevated, (read post about interpreting your TSH test). In the case of Graves' disease the TSH will be low. People with Hashimoto's and central hypothyroidism may have a normal reading on this test.

2. Thyroid peroxidase antibodies (TPO Antibodies) Thyroid peroxidase antibodies (TPO Antibodies) and Thyroglobulin Antibodies (TG Antibodies) – Most people with Hashimoto's will have an elevation of one or both of these antibodies. These antibodies are often elevated for decades before a change in TSH is seen. People with Graves' disease and

thyroid cancer may also have an elevation in thyroid antibodies including TPO & TG, as well as TSH receptor antibodies.

3. Thyroglobulin Antibodies (TG Antibodies) Read # 2

4. Thyroid Ultrasound Thyroid Ultrasound – A small percentage of people may have Hashimoto's, but may not have thyroid antibodies detectable in the blood. Doing a thyroid ultrasound will help your physician determine a diagnosis.

5. Free T3 Free T3 & Free T4 – These tests measure the levels of active thyroid hormone circulating in the body. When these levels are low, but your TSH tests in the normal range, this may lead your physician to suspect a rare type of hypothyroidism, known as central hypothyroidism.

6. Free T4

7. Reverse T3

You must be an advocate for health and insist on all the following tests especially the two thyroid antibody tests.

Thyroid Peroxidase Antibodies (TPOAb) #2

Thyroglobulin Antibodies (TgAb) #3

Don't allow your doctor to refuse to give you these tests. Many people have normal lab tests but still have Hashimoto's disease. It's all in the antibodies!

Disclaimer:

Readers are urged to all appropriate precautions before taking on any "Do it yourself" task. Always follow the directions and use precautions when making your own homemade products. Never stretch your abilities to far. Each individual, fabric or material may react differently to particular suggested use. Although, this is a non-toxic and natural way to clean your home, always wear protective gloves and eye wear. Although every effort has been made to provide you with the best possible information, the publisher nor author are responsible for accidents, injuries, damage incurred as a result of tasks performed by readers. The author will not assume responsibility for personal or property damages from resulting in the use of formulas found in this book. This book is not a substitute for professional services.

The information and recipes contained in book are based upon the research and the personal experiences of the author. Every attempt has been made to provide accurate, up to date and reliable information. No warranties of any kind are expressed or implied. Readers acknowledge that the author is not engaging in the rendering of legal, financial, medical or professional advice. By reading this book and participating in the 21 day reboot program, the reader agrees that under no circumstance the author is not responsible for any loss, direct or indirect, which are incurred by using this information contained within this book. Including but not limited to errors, omissions or inaccuracies. This book is not intended as replacements from what your health care provider has suggested. The author is not responsible for any adverse effects or consequences resulting from the use of any of the suggestions, preparations or procedures discussed in this blog. All matters pertaining to your health should be supervised by a health care professional. I am not a doctor, or a medical professional. This book is designed for as an educational and entertainment tool only. Please always check with your health practitioner before taking any vitamins, supplements, or herbs, as they may have side-effects, especially when combined with medications, alcohol, or other vitamins or supplements. Please check with you health care provider to see if you can do the 21 day reboot whereas you might have other health conditions that will not allow you to. Knowledge is power, educate yourself and find the answer to your health care needs. Wisdom is a wonderful thing to seek. I hope this book will teach and encourage you to take leaps in your life to educate yourself for a happier & healthier life. You have to take ownership of your health.

A.L. Childers

Copyrighted Material

Copyright 2017 Audrey Childers.

This book, or parts thereof, may not be reproduced in any form without the written permission from the Author. All rights reserved. This book is copyright protected. You cannot sell, distribute, use, quote or paraphrase any part or the content within this book without of the author. Legal action will be pursued if breached.

All rights reserved. In accordance with the U.S. write copyright act of 1976, the scanning, the uploading, and electronic scanning of any part of this book. Without permission of the publisher or author constitutes unlawful piracy and theft of the author's intellectual property. If you would like to use material from this book. (Other than for review purposes), prior written permission must be obtained by contacting the author @ permissions @ audreychilders@hotmail.com. Thank you for your support of the author's rights.

Thanks for reading my latest book. Please let me know if you need any support with it.

A note of caution:

I strongly support self-care, personal health empowerment and improving your understanding of thyroid health. However, this cannot substitute by a trained medical professional in cases of long standing and undiagnosed symptoms. This book is thus not meant as a substitute for professional medical judgement, though it can serve as a helpful adjunct to it. All content within this book is commentary or opinion and is protected under Free Speech laws in all the civilized world. The information herein is provided for educational and entertainment purposes only

When in doubt about your thyroid seek your doctor or your medical professional to exclude serious medical conditions. It is not intended as a substitute for professional advice of any kind. Audrey Childers assumes no responsibility for the use or misuse of this material.

Therefore no warranty of any kind, whether expressed or implied, is given in relation to this information. This is a comprehensive limitation of liability that applies to all damages of any kind, including (without limitation) compensatory; direct, indirect or consequential damages; loss of data, income or profit; loss of or damage to property and claims of third parties.

Be safe, be sane and be healthy.

Get a complete exam from a reliable health practitioner. Do what you can do within the boundaries of good common sense.

In a word, be kind to yourself and your thyroid.

© Copyright Audrey Childers. All Rights Reserved.

Sources:

1) Asvold BO., "Thyrotropin levels and risk of fatal coronary heart disease: the HUNT study." Arch Intern Med. 2008 Apr 28;168(8):855-60.

2) Asvold BO., "The association between TSH within the reference range and serum lipid concentrations in a population-based study. The HUNT Study" Eur J Endocrinol February 1, 2007 156 181-186.

3) Baisier, W. V., "Thyroid Insufficiency. Is Thyroxine the Only Valuable Drug?" Journal of Nutritional & Environmental Medicine. (2001), 11, 159-166.

4) Carvalho, D. P., "Thyroid peroxidase activity is inhibited by amino acids" Brazilian Journal of Medical and Biological Research. 2000 Mar;33(3):355-61.

5) Fukusen N.,"Inhibition of chymase activity by phosphoglycerides." Archives of Biochemistry and Biophysics. 1985 Feb 15;237(1):118-23.

6) Chopra I.J., "Evidence for an inhibitor of extrathyroidal conversion of thyroxine to 3,5,3'-triiodothyronine in sera of patients with nonthyroidal

illnesses." The journal of clinical endocrinology and metabolism. 1985 Apr;60(4):666-72.

7) Tabachnick M., "Effect of long-chain fatty acids on the binding of thyroxine and triiodothyronine to human thyroxine-binding globulin." Biochimica et Biophysica Acta. 1986 Apr 11;881(2):292-6.

8) Wiersinga W.M., "Inhibition of nuclear T3 binding by fatty acids." Metabolism. 1988 Oct;37(10):996-1002.

9) Rafael J. "The effect of essential fatty acid deficiency on basal respiration and function of liver mitochondria in rats." The journal of nutrition. 1984 Feb;114(2):255-62.

10) Fery, F., "Hormonal and metabolic changes induced by an isocaloric isoproteinic ketogenic diet in healthy subjects." Diabetes and Metabolism. 1982 Dec;8(4):299-305.

11) Orzechowska-Pawiłojć, A., "The influence of thyroid hormones on homocysteine and atherosclerotic vascular disease" Endokrynol Pol. 2005 Mar-Apr;56(2):194-202.

12) Ramsden C.E., "Use of dietary linoleic acid for secondary prevention of coronary heart disease and death: evaluation of recovered data from the Sydney Diet Heart Study and updated meta-analysis." BMJ. 2013 Feb 4;346:e8707.

13) Shering, SG., "Thyroid disorders and breast cancer." Eur J Cancer Prev. 1996 Dec;5(6):504-6.

14) Ratcliffe, J. G.,"Thyroid function in lung cancer" Br Med J. Jan 28, 1978; 1(6107): 210–212.

15) Turken, O.,"Breast cancer in association with thyroid disorders." Breast Cancer Res. 2003;5(5):R110-3. Epub 2003 Jun 5.

16) Linos, A. "Does coffee consumption protect against thyroid disease?" Acta chirurgica Scandinavica. 1989 Jun-Jul;155(6-7):317-20.

17) Petrek, J.A., "The inhibitory effect of caffeine on hormone-induced rat breast cancer" Cancer. 1985 Oct 15;56(8):1977-81.

18) Nakanishi, N. "Effects of coffee consumption against the development of liver dysfunction: a 4-year follow-up study of middle-aged Japanese male office workers." Industrial Health. 2000 Jan;38(1):99-102.

19) Freedman, Neal D. "Association of Coffee Drinking with Total and Cause-Specific Mortality" New England Journal of Medicine. 2012; 366:1891-1904.

20) Nauman A., "The Effect of Adrenaline Pretreatment on the In Vitro Generation of 3,5,3'-Triiodothyronine and 3,3',5'-Triiodothyronine (Reverse T3) in Rat Liver Preparation" Hormone and metabolic research. 1984 Sep;16(9):471-4.

21) Heyma P., "Glucocorticoids decrease in conversion of thyroxine into 3, 5, 3'-tri-iodothyronine by isolated rat renal tubules." Clin Sci (Lond). 1982 Feb;62(2):215-20.

22) Laugero K.D., "A new perspective on glucocorticoid feedback: relation to stress, carbohydrate feeding and feeling better." J Neuroendocrinol. 2001 Sep;13(9):827-35.

23) Oarada M., "Fish oil diet affects on oxidative senescence of red blood cells linked to degeneration of spleen cells in mice." Biochim Biophys Acta. 2000 Aug 24;1487(1):1-14.

24) Herrero A., "Effect of the degree of fatty acid unsaturation of rat heart mitochondria on their rates of H2O2 production and lipid and protein oxidative damage." Mechanisms of ageing and development. 2001 Apr 15;122(4):427-43.

http://www.care2.com/greenliving/11-super-health-benefits-in-just-1-celery-stalk.html

http://draxe.com/benefits-of-celery/

http://healingthebody.ca/3-ingredients-to-watch-for-in-your-protein-powder/

Disclaimer

The information and recipes contained in this book are based upon the research and the personal experiences of the author. It's for entertainment purposes only. Every attempt has been made to provide accurate, up to date and reliable information. No warranties of any kind are expressed or implied. Readers acknowledge that the author is not engaging in the rendering of legal, financial, medical or professional advice. By reading this, the reader agrees that under no circumstance the author is not responsible for any loss, direct or indirect, which are incurred by using this information contained within this book. Including but not limited to errors, omissions or inaccuracies. This book is not intended as replacements from what your health care provider has suggested. The author is not responsible for any adverse effects or consequences resulting from the use of any of the suggestions, preparations or procedures discussed in this book. All matters pertaining to your health should be supervised by a health care professional. I am not a doctor, or a medical professional. This book is designed for as an educational and entertainment tool only. Please always check with your health practitioner before taking any vitamins, supplements, diet change, or herbs, as they may have side-effects, especially when combined with medications, alcohol, or other vitamins or supplements. Knowledge is power, educate yourself and find the answer to your health care needs. Wisdom is a wonderful thing to seek. I hope this book will teach and encourage you to take leaps in your life to educate yourself for a happier & healthier life. You have to take ownership of your health.

A.L. Childers

Copyrighted Material

Copyright 2016 Audrey Childers.

This book, or parts thereof, may not be reproduced in any form without the written permission from the Author. All rights reserved. This book is copyright protected. You cannot sell, distribute, use, quote or paraphrase any part or the content within this book without of the author. Legal action will be pursued if breached.

All rights reserved. In accordance with the U.S. write copyright act of 1976, the scanning, the uploading, and electronic scanning of any part of this book. Without permission of the publisher or author constitutes unlawful piracy and theft of the author's intellectual property. If you would like to use material from this book. (Other than for review purposes), prior written permission must be obtained by contacting the author @ permissions @ audreychilders@hotmail.com. Thank you for your support of the author's rights.

Thanks for reading my latest book. Please let me know if you need any support with it.

I would like to thank you for taking the 1st steps in a journey to renew your health. Diet does have a direct affect way in which the body absorbs thyroid medication. You should always discuss with your doctor any dietary changes. We need to change the way we eat. Change the chemicals we use on our bodies, change the chemicals we use in our homes, read labels and ask questions. Eat foods that are rich in nutrients and minerals like veggies and fruits, and make a choice to avoid artificial flavors, additives and ingredients. For more tips, recipes, non-toxic household cleaning & body recipes on Kicking Hypothyroidism booty please follow me on twitter @thyroidismchick , @thyroidismchick on Instagram. Please follow my blog Thehypothyroidismchick.com. Where I send out weekly blogs and newsletters with the latest and greatest recipes, tips and idea's directly in your inbox! My mission is to do everything in my power to help you reach your fullest potential. Be the source of inspiration you seek and captivate what you relish with faith, that your vision of victory is your own kismet.